THE
WALKING MED

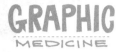

Susan Merrill Squier and Ian Williams,
General Editors

Editorial Collective
MK Czerwiec (Northwestern University)
Michael J. Green (Penn State University College of Medicine)
Kimberly R. Myers (Penn State University College of Medicine)
Scott T. Smith (Penn State University)

Books in the Graphic Medicine series are inspired by a growing awareness of the value of comics as an important resource for communicating about a range of issues broadly termed "medical." For healthcare practitioners, patients, families, and caregivers dealing with illness and disability, graphic narrative enlightens complicated or difficult experience. For scholars in literary, cultural, and comics studies, the genre articulates a complex and powerful analysis of illness, medicine, and disability and a rethinking of the boundaries of "health." The series includes original comics from artists and non-artists alike, such as self-reflective "graphic pathographies" or comics used in medical training and education, as well as monographic studies and edited collections from scholars, practitioners, and medical educators.

Other titles in the series:

MK Czerwiec, Ian Williams, Susan Merrill Squier, Michael J. Green, Kimberly R. Myers, and Scott T. Smith, *Graphic Medicine Manifesto*

Ian Williams, *The Bad Doctor: The Troubled Life and Times of Dr. Iwan James*

Peter Dunlap-Shohl, *My Degeneration: A Journey Through Parkinson's*

Aneurin Wright, *Things to Do in a Retirement Home Trailer Park: . . . When You're 29 and Unemployed*

Dana Walrath, *Aliceheimers: Alzheimer's Through the Looking Glass*

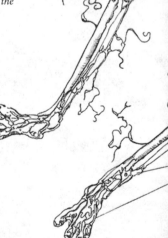

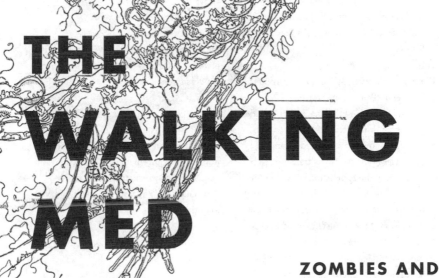

THE
WALKING
MED

ZOMBIES AND

THE MEDICAL IMAGE

Edited by

Lorenzo Servitje and Sherryl Vint

Foreword by Steven Schlozman

THE PENNSYLVANIA STATE UNIVERSITY PRESS
UNIVERSITY PARK, PENNSYLVANIA

Library of Congress Cataloging-in-Publication
Data

Names: Servitje, Lorenzo, 1983– , editor. |
    Vint, Sherryl, 1969– , editor.
Title: The walking med : zombies and the
    medical image / edited by Lorenzo Servitje
    and Sherryl Vint ; foreword by Steven
    Schlozman.
Other titles: Graphic medicine.
Description: University Park, Pennsylvania :
    The Pennsylvania State University Press,
    [2016] | Series: Graphic medicine | Includes
    bibliographical references.
Summary: "Shows how our understanding of
    narratives of illness can by transformed by
    recognizing the zombie metaphors within
    them and how the recent medicalization of
    popular zombie narratives has added new
    dimensions to what is symbolized by this
    figure"—Provided by publisher.
Identifiers: LCCN 2016025161 | ISBN
    9780271077116 (cloth : alk. paper) | ISBN
    9780271077123 (pbk. : alk. paper)
Subjects: | MESH: Cartoons as Topic | Ethics,
    Medical | Attitude of Health Personnel |
    Medicine in Art | Medicine in Literature |
    United States
Classification: LCC R733 | NLM WZ 336 |
    DDC 610—dc23
LC record available at https://lccn.loc.gov/
    2016025161

CON-TENTS

FORE-WORD

Steven Schlozman

In the complex world of medicine and culture, zombies wear many hats. To that end, my response to this wonderful collection of provocative and admittedly sometimes unsettling essays is based on which of my own professional hats I happen to be wearing.

As a practicing physician, I admit that I am simultaneously excited and unnerved. My entire training is predicated on the largely Western and perhaps especially American notion that health is itself a binary prospect. That's the way our reimbursement system works. You are either well or you are ill. You are either sick or you are healthy. It is as if we learned to be doctors in preparation for the digital world of ones and zeros that has come to dominate our entire social landscape. And yet here, in this book, we discuss murky concepts such as "living cadavers" and us/them mergers. Zombies aren't just ravenous, shambling ghouls. They are uncomfortably recognizable symbols of economic and racial inequalities. If these kinds of notions don't bring to mind our maddening healthcare system, then you haven't been reading the news. The American healthcare system may in fact be the tail that wags the dog of how we practice. We define sickness by that which is remunerated. Clinicians are reimbursed most often for recognizing sickness, so as a culture we fail to carefully elucidate health. This is akin to the now wildly familiar theme of a zombie outbreak forcing the unafflicted survivors to become paradoxically less human. We are increasingly clumsy at appreciating the spaces *in between*. The irony here is that our improving technical prowess in medicine means that the boundaries between self (healthy) and Other (sick) are more and more blurred. Still, we cling to our staked-out poles.

Enter graphic medicine. Colors and appearances and even the tone of the speakers in both fictional and nonfictional narratives can express these nuances better than any electronic medical record can.

The same line of thought emerges if I change my hat and put on instead my medical-educator derby. My students have been taught that there are specific criteria that make somebody sick. In fact, I have taught them those criteria. High blood pressure is a number—a measurement that is exactly quantifiable—that reflects the pressure with which blood pushes against the walls of the body's precious vasculature. Similarly, as a psychiatric educator, I have taught my students that two weeks of neurovegetative symptoms signals an entity called depression, but that less than two weeks means we ought to hesitate with that signifier. We don't, of course, tell our students to ignore the patient whose blood pressure is "normal" but who has symptoms of hypertension. Neither do we instruct our students that the suicidal patient who has felt this way for less than two weeks is somehow less seriously suffering. But we struggle in the educational sphere with these gray areas, because our students do not, as a rule, relish this kind of ambiguity. To be fair, neither does the rest of our culture. The strength of the zombie narrative rests in its ability to make us directly face these ambiguities. As a rule, it is a disorienting and terrifying moment in a zombie film when someone must decide if what used to be family is now not even human. The subtle and intellectually stimulating distinctions inherent in blurred pathological gradations are often lost in these moments of a zombie story, and they are similarly lost among those medical students whose concern is, understandably, whether what they are being asked to learn will later show up on a multiple-choice test.

Again, graphic medicine comes to my rescue. I can imagine, and indeed I have already made use of the imagery and tone of this kind of exercise, as a means of making available those very nuances that seem to otherwise elude the lecture hall or the teaching bedside.

But I have one more hat to wear in this discussion.

I have written a medically themed, graphically illustrated, and only barely tongue-in-cheek zombie novel. If I were a narcissistic guy (and I've already used way more personal pronouns than is typically acceptable), I might be tempted to think that I have inspired some of the complex and complicated notions that we've explored in this book.

Regardless of whether I play a role in this movement, I do in fact take great solace in these essays. By reading these chapters and digesting (if you'll pardon the zombie pun) the material, I have—appropriate enough to the aims of graphic medicine—realized what I rather suspected all along but could not quite get into words. The zombie metaphor, in both literature and medicine, has been fueled by a sneaky and impressive profundity. When my wife tells me that I am becoming a zombie myself as I indulge in one zombie story after another, I can now turn (as will many readers, I'd hazard) to this very book and say, "Wrong, my dear!" By watching these films and reading these stories and digesting all that these tales have to say, I am paradoxically avoiding the mindless traps that the zombie has set for me.

In other words, I am resisting zombification by indulging in it. If ever there were a postmodern epiphany, this would be it. I think about zombies and therefore I am not a zombie. And, if this is the case, then the converse must be true. By *not* thinking about zombies, I risk mindlessly consuming whatever I am fed. This book can be a catalyst for whatever might cure our broken and rigid world. This is perhaps especially salient when it comes to modern medicine.

I am aware that this sounds grandiose, but allow me at least to make my point in a realm of now-familiar tropes. What if medicine itself is the real zombie? What if our current system of care, with its faceless and deadened doctors and depersonalized insurance prior authorizations and emphasis on randomized controlled trials at the expense of actual connection, is the most relevant and pressing embodiment of the walking dead in our everyday lives? *Remember that the strength of the zombie story—the very core of zombie horror—is that zombies don't care.* Hungry zombies find nothing special about your intestines. A zombie would just as soon eat the next guy's intestines. Your intestines aren't great but they're also not *not* great. They're just intestines—the same as the next guy's. Do you see what I'm saying? To the zombie gastroenterologist your colon is the same as the next colon . . . just one more colonoscopy. That's a far cry from the sentiment that medical students express in their personal essays when they apply to medical school.

Of course I'm being deliberately glib. Doctors are still doing their best to be caring. Physicians are still doing their best to treat their patients as unique and special. But you need only visit an emergency ward or a waiting room to sense the growing despair in both patient and doctor alike. Sometimes the system seems so broken that the doctors themselves become numb. They shuffle around in white coats, ushering patients through real or imagined revolving doors; and though we still receive impressive and even miraculous care from scientific and technical expertise, it is increasingly rare to find the physician who is not to some extent zombified by the process.

Here's where graphic medicine can be particularly useful. In fact, this is where any form of artistic displacement in thinking about medicine can perhaps allow us to resist the systemic pandemic of zombified medicine.

Graphic medicine removes us just enough from the fray that we can actually pay attention. A picture or a comic doesn't ooze into the next frame the way rapid patient encounters ooze into one another. The picture in a comic exists as a unique entity and demands to be seen. George Pfau's haunting artwork is a perfect example. How do we maintain our humanity and thus resist the self/Other dichotomies that are surely oversimplifications of what it means to be a physician or patient? As Ringo Starr told us almost fifty years ago, it don't come easy.

As this book demonstrates, zombies provide the perfect metaphor for what *not* to do. Remember that zombies, once zombies, *don't know* they're zombies. A broken medical world might not recognize that it is broken if the break is pandemic and omnipresent. So we must learn to recognize the precursors to the metaphoric zombie medical plague before it happens. And we learn how to do this through teaching medicine from a different point of view. That allows us to see what we might become before we go into the world and become it.

I've taught medical students with PowerPoint images of human sagittal brain transections, and with the same depictions but this time of a putative zombie. Do you have to guess which image grabs their attention?

But that's just the attention grabber. That's like Shaun in the zombie film *Shaun of the Dead* (Edgar Wright 2004). A good part of the fun of that movie is the viewer's simultaneous ability to witness all the signs of impending doom that Shaun fails to notice and at the same time to appreciate how the drudgery of Shaun's life prevents him from taking note of his increasingly alarming surroundings. But Shaun's taking note of the mess he's in is the prelude to his finally taking action. In a similar fashion, the real lesson comes in asking those students why they notice *more* with a drawn and fictional image than with the real thing. And then we hit them with the zombie zinger—is a person suffering from zombiism a person at all? According to the trope, the answer is no. But if you're a doctor, then that can *never* be your answer. A person is a person is a person. Sick or well or dead or alive or any of the spaces in between, that person is still human.

That's the gift of the zombie to medicine.

PREF-ACE

Lorenzo Servitje and Sherryl Vint

The Zombie Turn

Over the last ten to fifteen years, popular culture has embraced the figure of
the zombie with an enthusiasm that few would have predicted in the years
before this zombie craze. Once of interest to only a subcultural group of
dedicated horror fans, zombies have moved from the pages of *EC Horror*
comics and the screens of midnight cult cinema to become the focus of major
Hollywood productions such as *World War Z* (Marc Forster 2013) and prof-
itable cable series such as AMC's *The Walking Dead* (2010–) comic adaptation, one of the highest rated and most syndicated television dramas at this
moment of writing. So, why zombies and why now? What drives and shapes
the recent cultural obsession with the meanings of this abject figure?

The zombie as currently understood is a relatively recent cultural invention. Both Sarah Lauro (2015) and Roger Luckhurst (2015), in their recent
cultural histories of the zombie, trace the process through which anxieties
about rebellious slaves and colonial fantasies of indigenous cannibalism
fused to transform the African and Haitian folklore figure of the *zombi* into
the American popular culture's image of the zombie as flesh-eating monster.
Folkloric *zombis* are abject figures returned from the dead and enslaved to
a master, and they were first introduced to American culture via William
Seabrook's sensationalist travel narratives, most famously adapted in the
Hollywood films *White Zombie* (Victor Halperin 1932) and *I Walked with a
Zombie* (Jacques Tourneur 1943). Oppressed by exploitative masters, these
zombies were more wretched than terrifying figures, objects of pity as much
as horror. Crucially, as Luckhurst argues, before the Second World War the
zombie was predominantly an individual, dehumanized victim rather than
a creature that appears only collectively as a mass. Zombies are the déclassé

cousins of more aristocratic monsters such as the vampire, within more recent history, even in their folkloric variant, a "distinctly modern contribution" to Gothic traditions that embody the monstrous: zombies are "products of our industrial modernity" (Luckhurst 2015, 10).

As Lauro's work in particular makes clear, zombies also function as something like a return of the repressed for colonizing cultures, all the violence of the imperial enterprise brought home to the domestic space. Their vacant stares, exhausted shuffles, and enthralled will provide a living specter of the destruction of slavery and its violent extraction of labor. Following Orlando Patterson's work on slavery as a kind of social death, both Lauro and Luckhurst argue that the *zombi* is both an embodiment of the violence done by slavery and a figure of violent resistance to such exploitative regimes. The pathologization of voodoo and the popularization of the abject figure of the zombie, they remind us, emerge from a history of colonial oppression in Haiti in which local spiritual community and beliefs often formed the backbone of collective resistance to slavery and ongoing colonization, both territorial and economic. Although the more recent popular culture image of the zombie largely ignores this early history, traces of it remain. Indeed, the recent shift in texts that begin to sympathize with rather than flee zombies and zombification—such as Isaac Marion's novel *Warm Bodies* (2011) and Jonathan Levine's film adaptation of the same (2013); or the British television series *In the Flesh* (2013–14)—reactivate some of this history of the zombie as a figure of our own potential subjugation. The phenomenon of zombie walks, some of which include zombie-themed bridal parties, demonstrate that the more the zombie craze continues, the more the zombie is seen as "us" rather than as "Other." Indeed, Lauro (2015, 77) suggests that the zombie may become the ground for a critical rethinking of human identity because "at its most basic level the living dead zombie represents a defiance of the binary categories imposed by Enlightenment reason, many of which, like the self/Other distinction, undergird capitalism."

The zombie mythos began a transformation in the post-WWII period, and Luckhurst (2015) argues that such changes were motivated in part by shifts in warfare, from the images of skeletal and seemingly living-dead victims of concentration camps, to the unfathomable destructiveness of the atomic bombs dropped on Japan, to the technique of using a "human wave" of troops treated as expendable to overcome antagonists with superior military technology during the Korean War. While not precisely zombies, such images, Luckhurst argues, pushed the zombie figure toward new associations as contemporary culture sought to come to terms with "the *massification* of death" (114). The turning point of the current and massively popular image of the zombie, however, came a bit later, with George Romero's *Night of the Living Dead* (1968). As Luckhurst is careful to point out, it is not until this film becomes the foundation for a franchise that the word "zombie" begins to be attached to its monstrous creatures, but nonetheless *Night* establishes many of the tropes that are now common in recent zombie texts: the transformation of loved humans into dangerous Others, and thus the need to immediately cease treating them as human; the idea that zombification is the result of some kind of contamination that is contagious (in this case, from space; later, viral); the fact that the more dangerous threat often comes from other humans, either those incapable of adjusting to the new situation or those seeking to exploit it to their own advantage; and finally the complete irrelevance of traditional humanist values, such as community or empathy or even family, in the face of the zombie apocalypse.

The dominant critical response to the current zombie obsession focuses on the way the zombie narrative encapsulates the vicissitudes of life under neoliberalism. In such readings, the erosion of any values beyond those of basic survival at any cost is seen to emblematize the dismantling of the welfare state under the rhetoric of necessity and economic crisis. Much like love or generosity are nostalgic fantasies that jeopardize one's survival in a zombie apocalypse, so, too, it would seem, do things such as social safety nets, mandated living wages, and the like threaten the health of "the economy," which has come to stand in for society. Henry Giroux's (2010) *Zombie Politics and Culture in the Age of Casino Capitalism* and Chris Harman's (2009) *Zombie Capitalism: Global Crisis and the Relevance of Marx* exemplify this approach, which is also evident in a number of readings of specific zombie texts. Indeed, so dominant has this approach become that a recent *Time* editorial pronounced zombies "the official monster of the recession" (Grossman 2009). Such economic and political readings of the zombie participate in a longer history of literary monsters serving to help us work through the alienation of capitalist extraction of surplus labor, as David McNally (2011) outlines in *Monsters of the Market*, making visible a traumatic violence of exploitation that began with land enclosures in the early modern period. The world of laborers whose physical bodies but not human subjectivities are required by capital parallels the subjectivity produced by what Achille Mbembe (2003, 21), discussing the nonhuman status of slaves, calls necropolitics, where the subject is "kept alive but in *a state of injury*, in a phantom-like world of horrors and intense cruelty and profanity." The image of the zombie horde reveals the way that the working classes are regarded as dehumanized and expendable, and it is only in our contemporary period—when such precarity is widely shared—that the zombie has moved from a marginal to central place in our cultural imagination.

The project of this book, then, is to build on this history of the zombie's meanings and to consider what new things it might signify in the context of contemporary for-profit healthcare, dehumanized working conditions including those among healthcare workers, and biomedical protocols that seem to blur the lines between the living and the dead. These histories of the *zombi* as figure of enslavement and rebellion, and of the zombie as disenfranchised and exploited labor, remain relevant, but new meanings also accrue if we shift the zombie into the terrain of medical humanities. The mythos itself has already moved in this direction, the crucial text being Danny Boyle's film *28 Days Later* (2003), in which zombies are a result of neither occult practices nor alien infestation, but are rather the unintended result of biomedical experimentation on the "rage virus" in weapons research. The zombie here moves from living dead to infected living, a transition that has influenced texts that follow, alongside Boyle's other innovation, the transformation of zombies from slow and shuffling to fast and rabid. Even recent texts that retain the slow-moving and corpse-like zombies, such as *The Walking Dead*, still adopt this medical reframing: zombification is a viral disease that affects all who die.

Luckhurst also points to another and earlier medical context that is important to the rethinking of zombies from the date of Romero's *Night of the Living Dead* until now: the legal production of the new category of brain death—an early term for such patients was "living cadaver"—to describe patients with "a complete absence of cortical activity . . . but who continued to live on within the biotechnical apparatus of the ICU" (175). This new medical classification produced a paradoxical subject that was a human body yet not to be treated as a human patient, such as in the case of harvesting organs for transplant. This was only the first of a by-now legion series of biomedical subjects that challenge our conceptual boundaries between living and dead, human and nonhuman, such as fertilized but frozen embryos unused in IVF procedures, immortal cell lines used in research, or aborted fetuses used as a source of stem cells. Bioethicists struggle to understand and respond to these novel biomedical subjects and contexts, and it is clear that the zombie, with its legacy of standing in for the dehumanized and abjected, can convey some of these ethical stakes in thinking through new regimes of living and dying.

Finally, and most obviously, the recent image of the zombie as figure of contagion speaks to our ongoing fears of global pandemic and to recent outbreaks that have demonstrated how quickly widespread contagion could overwhelm social structures. The pyres of burning animals in response to SARS, for example, echo the postapocalyptic landscapes of most zombie texts. The moral and other panics that emerge in response to a threat of contagion—which often represent the potentially infected as dangerous antagonists rather than as human beings in need of medical help—are informed by and further reinforce the harsh logic of zombie tales of survivalism. As if the virus itself were taking cues from zombie texts, the recent Ebola outbreak revealed that this virus can live on past the host's death, making dead bodies a dangerous source of contagion (Luckhurst 2015, 182). As is frequently noted, the fear that we have become dehumanized by the experience of trauma and our response to perceived threat is a ubiquitous theme of contemporary zombie narratives, and they may find their echo in responses to real outbreak crises. This history dates as far back as the AIDS crisis, Luckhurst points out, citing an early news article, written at a time when AIDS was still understood as a "Haitian disease," that used the language of the "living dead" to describe its sufferers, neatly linking contemporary zombies back to their *zombi* progenitors. The CDC recently produced a graphic novel about zombies, and in the UK the Wellcome Trust more recently used a similar model in its Glasgow-based Zombie Institute for Theoretical Studies (9). Such examples show that even medical practitioners recognize the parallels between the reinvention of zombie mythology in the twenty-first century and the contemporary threat of contagion.

The CDC's comic book project is our point of entry for the critical project of this book, which is to put this cultural work of analyzing the zombie mythos into dialogue with recent work in medical humanities that sees the comic book form as a crucial educational and ethnographic tool. We will discuss in more detail below how putting these two communities of scholars in dialogue produced the at-times surprising research collected here, but first we need to turn from the context of cultural meanings of zombies to introduce the emergent field of graphic medicine.

Graphic Medicine

Graphic medicine is defined by "the interaction between the medium of comics and the discourse of healthcare" (Squier and Marks 2014, 145). As an expanding field of research and practice it has come into view in mainstream academic research, such as the publication of Michael Green's (2013) comic

"Missed It" in the *Annals of Internal Medicine* and the dozens of citations of Green and Myers's (2010) publication on the use of comics in healthcare, the first of its kind, in the *BMJ*. More recently, Ian Williams's memoir *The Bad Doctor* and MK Czerwiec, Michael Green, Ian Williams, Susan M. Squier, Kimberly Myers, and Scott Smith's (2015) *Graphic Manifesto* were enthusiastically received in the *New York Times*. Much of the work in graphic medicine has focused on autobiographical texts pertaining to illness, what Green and Myers (2010) call "graphic pathographies." These graphic texts and their readings often take the form of challenging clinical norms and interrogating the limitations of medical intervention and its practitioners (Cole 2012). For instance, Squier (2008) reads the graphic novels *Epileptic* (2006) and *The Ride Together: A Brother and Sister's Memoir of Autism in the Family* (2004) as medium-specific texts that disrupt and challenge the presumed categories of normalcy and disability (2). Ian Williams (2014) cites a number of well-known and influential texts in the field and argues that medicine has influenced "comics," not only in how the medium reflects illness and but also in shaping how illness is perceived and conveyed through what Sander Gilman calls "the iconography of illness." The range of the comics in earlier conceptions of graphic medicine tended to fall between patients' (and their family members') graphic pathographies and medical practitioners' experience in providing care.

Williams (2015, 123) suggests that graphic pathographies can play a role in creating alternate schematic productions because they might help us rethink the discourse of health and social mediation of illness beyond the clinic. Squire (2015, 51–52) makes a similar argument, considering Kirsten Ostherr's biocultural studies of biomedicine with respect to visual culture, suggesting that comics are a powerful medium to broaden the audience of health humanities and related scholarship. We would second this contention, adding that we can perhaps augment our audience beyond researchers even more by adopting the seemingly contagious popular culture figure of the zombie—a tactic that many biomedical researchers are already using, as discussed further the introduction to this volume. Like Ostherr's (2013) notion that the cultural appropriations of medical films and visual culture influenced medical practice, authors in this volume observe "what happens" when biomedical researchers and practitioners take up the popular culture figure of the zombie in the visual culture of comics and graphic novels.

What makes this field so productive is the way it attracts a diverse group of perspectives, in terms of research and scholarship—literary, comics, and academic medicine scholars—but also in terms of the medical profession—nurses, doctors, medical students, and other actors in medical care, from patient to professional. Beyond the medical professionals, graphic medicine as a field includes medical illustrators and biomedical communication researchers who have become key participants in the field, such as Shelly Wall (2016) and Lydia Gregg. Following this trajectory, we move beyond comics and graphic pathographies to take an interest in the relevance of medical illustration and its history to this intersection of zombie mythology and graphic medicine. Although its practitioners have been involved in graphic medicine, the role of medical illustration has been in sufficiently analyzed. We want to think about how zombie images that draw on medical illustration work within and as medical narratives. To this end, we look at traditional graphic novels and comics but also beyond them.

The Walking Med is a response to Williams's (2012, 27) call to evaluate what kinds of graphic texts should be included within the cannon of illness narratives. It proposes a critical examination of the ubiquitous zombie figure vis-à-vis medical discourse and medical humanities in visual "texts." Comics are more formally characterized as "sequential art," a term commonly deployed in scholarly work on graphic medicine and often citing the work of Will Eisner (2008) and Scott McCloud (1994). In this volume we want to expand what counts as graphic medicine. We consider graphic texts in continuum with medical illustration to expand the ways science and technology studies (STS), biomedical communications, art, medical history, and visual culture more broadly can enrich the study and practice of graphic medicine. As the field that is still emerging and defining its scope, what graphic medicine will become is contingent on new and diverse conversations.

The Volume

This volume brings together two communities of scholars who had not previously been in dialogue: those working on the cultural meanings of zombies, as discussed in the first section above, and those working in the field of graphic medicine, described in the second section of this preface. This was a challenging project, but we think the results are exciting and useful to both fields of study. Many of our contributors were surprised when we asked them to think about their work in this context: those accustomed to analyzing the cultural meanings of zombies saw this figure as predominantly informed by the histories of racial and class exclusion discussed above, while those working in graphic medicine did not readily see any zombies in the texts with which they worked. Indeed, while many—including ourselves—could think of many comic books that feature zombies, most of these did not, at least at first glance, seem overtly interested in questions of medicine and health; similarly, while the field of graphic medicine is premised on the combination of word and image to portray aspects of the experience of medical education and treatment, few seemed directly to use images of zombies, notwithstanding the zombie's popularity in contemporary culture, including popular images of contagion.

We persisted, however, because it seemed to us something needed examination at this nexus. Our experience in putting together this volume revealed to us the power of asking scholars to think in new ways as was required by the conjunction of zombies with graphic medicine. For the cultural studies scholars who theorize the zombie metaphor, being required to think of its relationship specifically with medicine enabled them to see new things about how the metaphor spoke to experiences of illness and the vulnerability of the ailing body, as the chapter by Gerry Canavan, in particular, points out. On the other side of the equation, asking medical practitioners and anthropologists to think about the zombie in relation to their work also revealed new ways to think about the experiences captured in the graphic narratives produced by their research subjects. When asked to look for images that fused zombies with medicine, our contributors were able to find them, and such images spoke powerfully to experiences of dehumanization, whether this be medical students fearing the erosion of their empathy, as Michael Green, Daniel George, and Darryl Wilkinson reveal, or cancer patients who feel their individuality is erased by the treatment protocol, as Juliet McMullin analyzes. The zombie metaphor does a specific kind of cultural work that allows novel perspectives to emerge within graphic medicine, and the dialogue between cultural studies and graphic medicine collected here enriches both fields.

A number of themes and motifs emerge across the chapters. A chief one is alienation, the experience of being less-than-human or invisible-as-human, which the zombie metaphor aptly captures. Given the zombie's history as a figure that emerged from the experiences of slavery and colonization, and then was revised to embody the traumas of mass slaughter in modern combat, it is striking that the zombie becomes visible as a predominant image of viral contagion in this cultural moment. The threat of a pandemic is linked to the same colonial histories of displacement, economic exploitation, and resource extraction from which the zombie emerged, now evident in the transnational flows of capital and commodities as vectors for contagion, or in the peculiar encounters between human and animal life produced by biotech and agribusiness. Steven Soderbergh's provocative film *Contagion* (2011) traces just these paths of neocolonial development as it reveals the origin of its zoonotic outbreak, and although it is not a zombie film its narrative of public panic and martial law in response to quarantine speaks to how strongly the zombie narrative shapes our sense of any outbreak. The more recent *World War Z* simply makes overt the zombie menace that haunts any outbreak narrative in this cultural moment, and similarly shows the confusion such events generate regarding whether they are evolved or engineered viruses, and also how those seen to be responsible for outbreak can be dehumanized in the response protocol.

Other essays point further, however, to the value of expanding the zombie metaphor beyond its obvious links to contagious disease. Both the Canavan and McMullin chapters are instructive here in helping us to see that the current zombie mania illuminates other aspects of public health crises as well. Although one does not typically think of zombies when one thinks of patients suffering from dementia, the parallels in impaired functionality are startling once one begins to think through this frame. Given the zombie's link to cultural analyses regarding the precariousness of contemporary life and work, it is useful to chart other kinds of diseases that might be shaped by and are in turn shaping recent zombie narratives. The image of the zombie brings to the surface connections between these particular experiences and other ways that the zombie has come to symbolize being outcast and expendable, helping us to see how certain populations—perhaps certain kinds of patients—are pathologized and to intervene in this process.

The process of compiling this volume points to directions for future research as well. For example, it seems to us productive to explore the degree to which the economic context in which the zombie has been read outside of graphic medicine intersects with a US-based medical culture rooted in profit. The scholarship collected here explores links between the marginality of certain kinds of economic subjects and the marginality of certain kinds of patients, and it would be fruitful for future research to think about how the for-profit healthcare system embodies and replicates for some the logic of apocalyptic survival at any cost that characterizes zombie texts. Finally, given the wealth of recent work in the medical humanities on how healthcare is influenced by legacies of systemic racism—combined with the zombie's history as a figure of racial marginalization—we think further research on this topic will also reveal additional insights to be gained by putting cultural studies of zombies and scholarship in graphic medicine into dialogue. This volume, then, begins a conversation rather than presents a comprehensive overview of this nexus. The insights collected here demonstrate what can be gained by pushing a cultural motif toward new associations and meanings and what can be learned by seeing graphic medicine's images within the larger field of popular culture.

Chapter Outlines

Rather than understanding the zombie as purely a manifestation or representation of medical, technological, and ecological anxieties, *The Walking Med* explores how the zombie is also transmuted and complicated in graphic texts. On the one hand, we see different aims and generic forms in the zombie's deployment, such as the CDC's public health zombie graphic novel—why did they not produce a short "viral" video, playing on the zombie film craze? On the other, we must consider difference in the effects produced by the medium: how does, for example, a patient's experience with terminal illness producing a feeling of "the undead" differ between a purely textual and a graphic story of illness? How does the combination of image and text help us come to terms with the liminal processes of brain death, as Margaret Lock would say, or the living death of chronic disease management? What, in short, can zombies signify in graphic medicine that they do not signify elsewhere and that is not otherwise representable within the field?

The volume opens with an introduction that examines the implications of bringing zombies into conversation with graphic medicine, where Lorenzo Servitje traces the uptake of the zombie metaphor in biomedical research and the emergence of "real zombies." Speaking to the mutual exchange between this research and popular culture, he cites the prominent case of *National Geographic*'s use of a comic to explain the ability of certain parasites to alter their hosts' behavior. Servitje suggests that there is a timeliness to research into the convergence of zombies, medicine, and graphic narratives, arguing that these intersections, demonstrated in the chapters that follow, can push graphic medicine toward new possibilities for research.

Our first section, "Diagnosing Zombie Culture," brings the interpretive work of cultural studies scholars to bear on the field of graphic medicine. These chapters read popular graphic fiction with an eye toward how they operate as critiques of medical cultures. Gerry Canavan explores how the zombie allegorizes aging and senescence in recent and less frequently discussed comic series such as *Revival* (2012–) and *Blackgas* (2007), in addition to the zombie inflections of Marvel and DC comics. Canavan links the threat of the zombie to the anxieties surrounding the ever-extended lifespan of the baby boomer generation. This is followed by Kari Nixon's treatment of how the authors of *The Walking Dead* (2003–) and *Crossed* (2008–10) exploit the liminal space of virality to question the binary constructions that sustain our modern medical and psychiatric enterprises. Ben Kooyman and Tully Barnett close this section with their examination of *The New Deadwardians*. They explore how the series depicts the abuse of medical knowledge and resulting social discontent, arguing that its use of zombie imagery suggests that the misuse and class stratification of medical assets is detrimental to and ultimately destroys both dominant and subordinate social strata, opening a space to critique the current status of Western medicine and society.

Taking the inverse approach to the first section, the chapters in "Reading the Zombie Metaphor" analyze texts from graphic medicine—medical and patient education, graphic pathographies, and so forth—and read them for their relevance to cultural studies of the zombie figure. Michael Green, Daniel George, and Darryl Wilkinson's chapter speaks to the recurring appearance of the zombie in comics drawn by fourth-year medical students in Green's "Comics and Medicine" seminar at Penn State College of Medicine, revealing what this figure suggests about the culture of medical education. Juliet McMullin conceptualizes "zombie toxins" in graphic cancer narratives to suggest that the zombie helps us understand the simultaneous exertions of life and death in the chemical regimes of chemotherapy treatments that disassemble bodies in order to save them. Sherryl Vint considers how the graphic adaption of Boyle's *28 Days Later* can be read against the narrative logic of the CDC's *Zombie Preparedness Guide*, suggesting that the former challenges the latter's rhetoric of confidence in medical authorities by opening a space to consider the complex human situations in which medicine actually happens.

The Walking Med closes with an unorthodox approach to graphic medicine in an effort to push the boundaries of the field beyond traditional sequential art in "Visualizing the Zombie Metaphor." These chapters interrogate how the zombie helps us to think about graphic medicine in dialogue with a longer history of the study of visual culture in medicine. Sarah Juliet Lauro opens this section, reading the zombie artwork of George Pfau (featured as a frontispiece in this volume) through recent scholarship in object-oriented ontology. Lauro demonstrates how Pfau's work draws on the history of anatomical illustration to conceptualize the way "Zombie Objects" reveal the laboring (after)lives of corpses and the subsequent ontological limits of defining a human body as thing versus as person. Lorenzo Servitje's chapter draws on the history of medical illustration to articulate how Steven Schlozman's illustrated novel *The Zombie Autopsies* (2011) critiques the objectivity of medical culture, specifically the diagnostic implications of recent STS research in neuroimaging. We conclude with Dan Smith's reading of Karen Green's *Lighter Than My Shadow*, which suggests that the graphic novel evokes the zombie not as a monstrous figure but rather as an embodiment of Giorgio Agamben's *Muselmann* to show how Green's *herstory* speaks to the biological and social boundaries of life and questions the ethics of witnessing such extreme conditions.

All our chapters reveal that thinking of the zombie in conjunction with the methodologies of graphic medicine is productive. This volume points toward further ways that the field of graphic medicine might grow as it continues a dialogue with the practices of cultural studies. We suggest that an investigation into the intersections of zombies and graphic medicine is a timely interdisciplinary convergence given the popular and biomedical interest in the figure. However, the implications of introducing the figure to graphic medicine will likely trump the zombie's popularity in terms of lasting effects. Scholars in graphic medicine are left with the questions of not only what to do with the zombie in graphic medical narratives—although we hope to have begun to answer some of those—but, more important, how to incorporate or reject the mythic and medical histories and the theoretical and methodological approaches the zombie brings with it.

REFERENCES

Czerwiec, MK, Michael Green, Ian Williams, Susan M. Squier, Kimberly Myers, and Scott Smith. 2015. *Graphic Medicine Manifesto.* University Park: Pennsylvania State University Press.

Eisner, Will. 2008. *Comics and Sequential Art: Principles and Practices from the Legendary Cartoonist.* New York: W. W. Norton.

Giroux, Henry A. 2010. *Zombie Politics and Culture in the Age of Casino Capitalism.* New York: Peter Lang.

Green, Michael J., and Kimberly R. Myers. 2010. "Graphic Medicine: Use of Comics in Medical Education and Patient Care." *BMJ: British Medical Journal (Overseas & Retired Doctors Edition)* 340 (7746): 574–77.

Green, Michael J., and Ray Rieck. 2013. "Missed It." *Annals of Internal Medicine* 158 (5): 357–61.

Grossman, Lev. 2009. "Zombies Are the New Vampires." *Time,* April 9. http://www.time.com/time/magazine/article/0,9171,1890384,00.html.

Harman, Chris. 2009. *Zombie Capitalism: Global Crisis and the Relevance of Marx.* London: Bookmarks.

Lauro, Sarah Juliet. 2015. *The Transatlantic Zombie: Slavery, Rebellion, and Living Death*. New Brunswick, NJ: Rutgers University Press.

Luckhurst, Roger. 2015. *Zombies: A Cultural History*. London: Reaktion Books.

Mbembe, Achille. 2003. "Necropolitics." Translated by Libby Meintjes. *Public Culture* 15 (1): 11–40.

McCloud, Scott. 1994. *Understanding Comics: The Invisible Art*. New York: Harper Perennial.

McNally, David. 2011. *Monsters of the Market: Zombies, Vampires, and Global Capitalism*. Leiden, NL: Brill.

Ostherr, Kirsten. 2013. *Medical Visions: Producing the Patient through Film, Television, and Imaging Technologies*. New York: Oxford University Press.

Squier, Susan. 2008. "So Long as They Grow out of It: Comics, the Discourse of Developmental Normalcy, and Disability." *Journal of Medical Humanities* 29 (2): 71–88.

———. 2015. "The Use of Graphic Medicine for Engaged Scholarship." In *Graphic Medicine Manifesto*, by MK Czerwiec, Michael Green, Ian Williams, Susan M. Squier, Kimberly Myers, and Scott Smith, 41–65. University Park: Pennsylvania State University Press.

Squier, Susan, and J. Ryan Marks. 2014. "Introduction." *Configurations* 22 (2): 149–52.

Wall, Shelly. 2016. "Comics in Clinical Education." In *Keeping Reflection Fresh: Top Educators Share Their Innovations in Health Professional Education*, edited by Allan Peterkin and Pamela Brett-MacLean. Kent, OH: Kent State University Press.

Williams, Ian. 2012. "Graphic Medicine: Comics as Medical Narrative." *Medical Humanities* 38 (1): 21–27.

———. 2014. "Graphic Medicine." In *Medicine, Health, and the Arts: Approaches to the Medical Humanities*, edited by Victoria Bates, Alan Bleakley, and Sam Goodman, 64–84. London: Routledge.

———. 2015. "Comics and the Iconography of Illness." In *Graphic Medicine Manifesto*, by MK Czerwiec, Michael Green, Ian Williams, Susan M. Squier, Kimberly Myers, and Scott Smith, 143–64. University Park: Pennsylvania State University Press.

GRAPHIC MEDICINE CONTRACTS THE ZOMBIE CRAZE:

An Introduction

Lorenzo Servitje

The approaches and methods that have emerged from the rapidly growing field of graphic medicine reveal new ways to think about how zombies draw from and shape biomedicine. In addition to looking at how zombie images and texts have appropriated medical tropes and narratives, it is worth both considering how "real medicine" has adopted the figure of the zombie as an explanatory metaphor and investigating the implications for graphic medicine. As we suggested in the preface to this volume, there has been a significant shift in the medicalization of the zombie figure, which has become understood through rubrics such as contagion, microbiology, and neuroscience. In this capacity it has become an important figure in shaping our current biomedicalized healthscape.[1] The biomedicalized zombie lends itself to medical humanistic approaches; moreover, the figure's pronounced presence in visual culture merits a new way of thinking about its relationship to biomedicine.

Enter graphic medicine: a field that continues to spur academic, pedagogical, and fan interest, growing into a substantial area of interdisciplinary research, especially in the medical/health humanities. Its most appealing quality is often cited as the way the juxtaposition of image and text creates a world of possibilities, as Ian Williams (2012, 25) suggests, for depicting the complexities, ambiguities, taboos, and absences of languages for disease, illness, and bodily sensations. With the zombie in mind, *The Walking Med* attends to these possibilities in comics and extends this to picture-and-word forms that are not strictly bound by that genre of "sequential art." Due in part to its ability to resist classification in the liminal state between life and death, subject and object, as Sarah Juliet Lauro and Karen Embry (2008) argue in their frequently cited article "A Zombie Manifesto," the zombie is a particularly productive figure to express and reflect on Williams's world of possibilities within human medical experience. The zombie compounds graphic medicine's ability to critique and theorize medical culture. As the authors of the *Graphic Medicine Manifesto* note, graphic medicine disrupts notions of techno-medical progress, universal patient experiences, and the dominant scholarly methods in healthcare (Czerwiec et al. 2015, 2–3). While a number of chapters in this volume address the zombie in terms of its more frequently identified tropes (plague, contagion, and epidemiology), other chapters move beyond identifying the similarities between the etiology of infectious disease and zombie plagues to question how medical discourse constructs and is constructed by popular iconography pertaining to the boundaries of life and death, illness and health. This introduction serves three aims: to think through the implications of using this language of the zombie in medical culture by considering how biomedical researchers utilize the figure of the zombie; to examine a case study of the visual zombie/medicine intersection in the case of zombie parasites; and, finally, to show how the zombie introduces perspectives from science and technology studies into graphic medicine, providing a richer way to think about figures such as the zombie within this emerging field.

Metaphors, Biomedicine, and "Real" Zombies

Like many tropes in science fiction, the zombie crosses discursive boundaries to become a metaphor used in clinical and scientific literature. As Michael Green, Daniel George, and Darryl Wilkinson note in their chapter on comics created by medical students, zombies are "good to think with." Because the zombie is so frequently identified as dehumanized figure, it is useful for conceptualizing patients who experience the "zombification" effects of illness and/or medical treatment, such as the numbing affect of clinical depression or ataxic effects seen in psychiatric patients who perform the "Thorazine shuffle"—a physical side effect that connotes more than the inability to ambulate properly and which has been read as a "zombie" symptom (Fhlainn

2011, 147). These are medicalized examples of the "cultural zombie," a non-literal figure of zombification engendered through its cultural milieu (Boon 2011, 8).

The popular press has a history of thinking of zombies in medical, specifically pharmacological frameworks. This can be traced at least as far back as the Canadian anthropologist Wade Davis's ethnobiological research on tetrodotoxin and tropane alkaloid intoxication with respect to zombification, what appears to be the first instance of an investigation of the "science" of reanimating the dead. His article in the *Journal of Ethnopharmacology* was excerpted in *Harper's* in 1984, and he went on to publish the highly popular *The Serpent and the Rainbow* (1985), which was later adapted to a film in 1988, now a cult classic, and *Passage: The Ethnobiology of the Haitian Zombie* (1988). Three decades later, the zombie was reintroduced to pharmacological discourse, this time strictly as metaphor. Since 2012 there has been a rash of "zombie" drugs reported in the news and popular media. The reports of psychosis-inducing bath salts, which resonated with the PCP "epidemic" of the late 1980s and 1990s, were frequently likened to zombies and zombie apocalypses.[2] In another instance, desomorphine has been characterized as a zombie drug due to its propensity to cause severe gangrene and necrosis, which manifests as decaying flesh falling off skulls and long bones. In the case of drugs it is clear that zombies, as figures of epidemics and societal threat, align with other medical metaphors such as the war on drugs and the war on infectious disease.

Drawing on the fascination for the epidemiological zombie, the Centers for Disease Control and Prevention made perhaps one of the most visible and publicized incorporations of zombies into biomedicine. In May 2011 the CDC generated headlines when it advised the public on how to prepare for a zombie apocalypse. "That's right, I said z-o-m-b-i-e a-p-o-c-a-l-y-p-s-e," writes Dr. Ali S. Khan on the CDC's *Public Heath Matters Blog* (2011), advising people how to stock up on food, create emergency kits, and become familiar with evacuation routes. They went on to publish a full-length digital graphic novel in which the authors adopt the common viral narrative of zombie contagion and label the pathogen "Z5N1," resonating with the panic surrounding avian flu or H5N1 (Silver et al. 2011). Here, the zombie most obviously and explicitly stands in for the emergency preparedness for any public health emergency.

According to some biomedical research, however, zombies are not so much metaphorical as they are very a "real" phenomena—this, of course, depends on what you mean by *zombie*. In the case of zombies being the dead come back to life, they are purely fictional. If, however, zombies are defined by the older denotation, as an organism "enslaved" through a form of behavior or "mind" control, there are two ways this can actually occur: drugs, as in the case cited by Wade Davis, and parasites. However, before explaining these "real" zombies, I would like to consider the significance of the fact that scientific research has taken an interest in making such claims.

A brief bibliometric analysis illustrates the degree to which biomedical culture has appropriated the zombie figure as a metaphor, an object of study, or in some cases both.[3] Before 1990 there were eight biomedical publications that reference the term *zombie*, two of which were directly discussing the case of tetrodotoxin and tropane alkaloid poisoning in Haiti either by Wade Davis or by those discussing his findings. Between 1990 and 2010 eighteen publications used the term. From 2010 to today there were thirty-seven. Beginning with publications in 1990 the zombie came to mean a side effect from psychotropic drugs and/or cognitive dysfunction, with some exceptions. Though the use of the zombie for psychiatric and neurological discourses, such as Alzheimer's disease,[4] still remains a common application,[5] the most prevalent usage from the early 2000s until today is linked to epidemics and parasitical relationships—namely, those where the "zombifying" parasite alters the host's behavior by hijacking the nervous system.[6] In 2013 the *Journal of Experimental Biology* ran a special issue (216, no. 1) on "Neural Parasitology." The *Journal of Integrative and Comparative Biology* followed a year later with its own issue, "Parasitic Manipulation of Hosts' Phenotype; or, How to Make a Zombie" (Weinersmith and Faulkes 2014). Some notable examples of this phenomenon include the jewel wasp, *Ophiocordyceps unilateralis* fungus, and the *gondii* species of toxoplasmosis. Interest in *Toxoplasmosa gondii* has extended outside of zoological parasitology, and researchers who study human behavior and psychiatric pathologies have developed theories which suggest that *T. gondii* may be a contributing factor in schizophrenia or other psychiatric conditions, in effect altering human behavior and personality by increasing the incidence of reckless choices (Flegr 2013).[7] Though these parasites have sparked some fears and sensation in the popular press about literal human zombification through infection and a "real" zombie apocalypse (Brune 2013), there are a number of practical and theoretical implications for studying such parasites beyond this "what if" scenario, such as new models of animal behavior for studying human affective disorders and novel understandings of how neurobiology alters behavior in contrast to the evolutionary nature of parasitic relationships (Adamo and Webster 2013, 1). We can relate this iteration of the zombie "slave" to current research that investigates how the microbiome influences behavior (Cryan and O'Mahony 2011). Consistent with the zombie's penchant for challenging binaries, these connections among the zombie, parasites, and neurology question monolithic and anthropocentric models of subjectivity.

The case of zombie parasites illustrates the very real influence that popular culture has on biomedicine. Although the zombifying parasites have been known to parasitologists and entomologists for some time, they have not been characterized by researchers *as such* until recently. Take *Ophiocordyceps unilateralis*, popularly known as "the zombie ant fungus," as an example. The fungus was discovered during the mid-Victorian period (Hughes et al. 2011); however, it was not until 2011 that researchers began to call the organism "the zombie ant fungus" in peer-reviewed publications, although popular Internet culture used the term as early as 2005.[8] These dates are not only temporally close to the resurgence of the zombie's popularity but also mark the period when the zombie becomes medicalized, discussed, and represented through epidemiological discourse and frequently following what Priscilla Wald (2008) calls "the outbreak narrative." While real-life epidemics do not always, and in fact rarely, have narrative components like a climax or resolution, the ways we think and talk about them do. As a figure of fiction that draws from some biomedical fact, the zombie is shaped by and shapes how we conceptualize the outbreak narrative. Even though the parasitic narrative draws on the older model of the voodoo-slave zombie, it does so through the trope of infection and contagion.

Considering this current conceptualization, especially the research on *T. gondii* and behavior, we can see that the slavery trope from the early twentieth century has not disappeared but instead has been displaced: from magic and voodoo to biology (Evans 2009). The nexus of the epidemiological "infectious" application of the zombie to the neurocognitive suggests that the plasticity of this figure to understand biomedical phenomena is both vast and resonant with contemporary culture. If medical educators are using zombies to teach neurobiology or, in the cases cited above, medical researchers are adopting the figure to explain parasites, the real/fictional binary is no longer a sufficient mode for describing the exchanges between culture and medicine.

Despite the fact that biomedicine increasingly looks toward a fantasy of permanent life extensions, zombie images and narratives are continual reminders that, in the case of brain-infecting parasites, our autonomous subjectivities are contingent and constructed. Moreover, because even their parasitological and epidemiological iterations more broadly still carry their earlier histories—in this case reanimated corpses—they underscore that death is permanently part of the state of life. Despite medical advances, "WE are the walking dead" (Kirkman, Moore, and Adlard 2005, issue 24). The zombie also reminds us of this inevitability and of the desires and technologies that seek permanently to forestall death—a central logic in our current biomedical moment of chronic disease management, with new specialties like geriatric and antiaging medicine, even the resurgent popularity of cryogenics. As Eric Cazdyn (2012, 2) writes, "The paradigmatic condition illustrating the already dead is that of the medical patient who has been diagnosed with terminal disease only to live through medical advances that then turn the terminal illness into a chronic one."[9]

These exposures and the problematization of these kinds of anxieties and preoccupations are well suited to the graphic medium through its specific capacity to bring forth what purely textual or purely visual and filmic narratives cannot fully articulate. As I have argued elsewhere (2015), the graphic medium invites and allows for extended reflection during narrative progression, a quality that film generally lacks. Furthermore, graphic texts can play with time in ways other mediums cannot. Susan Squier (2015, 51–53) notes that comics can represent time spatially in both diachronic and synchronic terms; they can capture both the traditional narrative time of illness and the "extralingustic," more difficult to express experiences of the temporality of illness. In these capacities we look to graphic texts, instead of film or television, to see the cultural work the zombie performs within medical discourse.

Graphic Parasitology

The cover of *National Geographic*'s November 2014 issue portrays an image of an insect that most educated readers would not recognize; however, the cover text labels this image with a term few would fail to recognize—"REAL ZOMBIES." The *National Geographic* story beautifully portrays via close-up photographs and detailed narratives the zombifying parasites previously mentioned. Each subsection dedicated to a particular parasite narrates the process of host zombification in comic form.

This use of a graphic narrative to explain an example of "real zombies" emblematizes precisely the kind of discursive intersection this book addresses and speaks to the timeliness of the chapters that follow. Let us return briefly to the zombic parasite, *T. gondii* or "toxo."

The particular mode and medium that *National Geographic* utilizes stands out. They have done a few comics in recent years but nothing with such a "graphic style," suggests artist and editor Matt Twombly. There is a common visual grammar in which parasitic relationships are usually presented to both scientific and general publics in everything from posters in veterinarian offices to biology textbooks, I suggest to Twombly in an e-mail exchange. He replies, "We wanted to do something fresh here, something that aligned with what inspired the photographer in his pictures. You're right, the typical life cycle diagram is some kind of circular flow chart, but that was too clinical for the mood we were trying to set. We wanted something eerie, with more appeal" (Twombly 2014). Consistent with the aims of graphic medicine as a practice and field of research, the reference to "setting the mood" speaks to the ability of the graphic medium to convey the affective dimensions of biomedical experience and understanding.

The short comic "The Case of the Fearless Rat" infuses the biological with the kind of affect produced in the horror genre—"something eerie"— like a zombie film. The grayscale color tones of the panels and title's font recall older horror films, specifically, I would suggest, George Romero's 1968 *Night of the Living Dead*. The circular panel, which simulates the microscopic view of the protozoa, keeps the microbiological process in the back of the reader's mind during the depicted interactions between rat, cat, and human, haunting the panels that follow. In other words, while we get an image of the zombified rat, clearly signaled by his colored eyes that stand out from the rest of the grayscale panel, we are encouraged think about how zombification is just a matter of scientific explanation rather than mythologized figures of Haitian slavery or reanimated corpses.

And yet the mood instilled by combination of panel, text, and narrative suggests that this phenomena, in contrast to a purely "scientific process," is like something out of a horror movie. The imperative here is not to inspire actual terror but to invoke the feeling of the genre in a somewhat playful capacity. When read closely, however, "The Case of the Fearless Rat" is more anxiogenic than it might first appear.[10] The final panel depicts the cat's presentation of the kill to his or her human. The text above reads, "Toxo can infect the brain of any mammal even humans," qualifying that statement by noting that it is rarely fatal but "can harm a pregnant woman's fetus"— the reason why pregnant women are often discouraged from handling cat litter (and, by extension, occasionally advised to avoid cats altogether). The following text reassures us, "Your cat is safe," as it cannot infect a feline's brain. The domestic imagery, though rural, brings the parasite home for readers, leaving them with questions that are implied by the images but left out of the text: Can it infect human brains? Can it alter human behavior? What does it do to *the children*? Related questions, as I noted above, are currently being asked and answered by researchers. The orange tint in the cat's eye recalls the mouse's eyes—along with the noxiously colored scent trail—and suggests a sinister influence. In this specific narrative we are left asking what happens next. Is that a female with the flats and rolled-up pant cuffs? *Is she pregnant?*

The zombie-parasite narrative leaves the reader to fill in the gaps—literally the gutters between panels—and the questions posed by the interaction between reader, text, and image. There is a certain immediacy to this visual that would not be present in a clinical life cycle image. The parasite-host relationship is dramatized to instill fear and curiosity, to delight as well as to educate. While it is not meant to be clinical in visual rhetoric, as the artist suggests, it does draw on and raise biomedical anxieties by capitalizing on the comic medium and the zombie narrative, on the zombie and the medical image. *National Geographic* illustrates how the zombie contributes to the public education in biomedical science through visual culture, in this case highlighting the cultural capital and value invested in the graphic form.

Conclusion

Science and technology studies (STS), media, and philosophy of science scholars have spoken to the centrality of visualization to scientific cultures and knowledge production, making them highly suitable for graphic medicine. For instance, Regula Valérie Burri and Joseph Dumit (2007) outline a representative variety of the approaches to the social study of scientific imaging and visualization. Dumit (2004) himself has done some of the seminal STS work specific to brain imaging, an approach I take up in my chapter in this volume. Lorraine Daston and Peter Galison (2007), in their landmark study of the shifting values in scientific epistemologies based on different modes of "seeing," explore the changes in the characteristics of scientific atlases from anatomical illustrations in the eighteenth century to the Visible Human Project and virtual renderings of nanotubules. They suggest that atlases, or scientific illustrations, "map" the sciences they serve and that they are the "systematic compilations" of "any manageable, communal representative of the sector of nature under investigation," what they call *working objects* (19–23). Lisa Cartwright (1995) traces the visual culture of medicine, in terms of optical techniques, cinematic media, and medical and popular images, to illuminate the ideological effects of the convergence of scientific and cultural practices in the visual medical idiom. More recently, Kirsten Ostherr (2013) investigates the way mass media like television has shaped what it means to be both a doctor and a patient by influencing clinical practice and the expectations of both sides of the medical equation.

The centrality of medicine's visual culture and the diverse actors responsible for medicine as a system of thought has practical implications for those in the medical field, as agents of its profession or as subjects under its care. Images of illness help structure the "schemata of illness" where the doctor creates and works within a differential mental catalog of signs and symptoms by which the next image or appearance of illness can be judged. For patients a similar logic holds true: they learn how to conceptualize and experience illness, building images of disease stereotypes (Williams 2015, 124). Since its emergence, scholarship in graphic medicine has sought to explore and complicate these schemas. Consequently, the introduction of the work of STS and visual culture scholars helps us see graphic medicine as part of a larger history of medicine as a visual culture—for example, as a kind of genealogical relative to medical illustration. Such connections put into question how different scientific histories and systems of thought inform the methods we use to illustrate medical experience and complicate its norms.

It is with this scholarship in mind that we turn to consider how the zombie figure reflects, produces, and critiques biomedical culture in graphic narratives and in less "orthodox" medical imagery and their accompanying text. The work of the authors in the volume builds on this established theory, bringing scholarship in medicine's visual culture along with critical and theoretical work surrounding zombies into the practice and scholarship of graphic medicine. And like the zombies' bidirectional exchange with medicine as a whole, *The Walking Med* more broadly develops a set of ways to think about both what graphic medicine brings to cultural studies and what cultural studies brings to graphic medicine.

The zombie as metaphor and figure does not appear ready to die anytime soon. If the past is any indication, however, it will certainly not remain static in either its visual or textual forms. Furthermore, the figure's shifting forms (from drugs, to viruses, to parasites) encourages us to continue to see the way it draws on popular and disciplinary understandings of biomedicine, revealing how medicine is "operating" beyond its biological intervention in the broader cultural sphere. But the zombie is only one such figure, and there is much more of this kind of work to be done. Graphic medicine clearly lends itself to such an endeavor.

NOTES

1. Adele Clarke and colleagues (2010) classify the period after 1985 as the era of biomedicalization, where changes in technoscience, political economy, and biopolitics shaped a new landscape for medical culture in practice, research, and public culture, with optimization being one of the imperatives engendered in this new era.
2. See Seitz-Wald (2013). This no doubt inspired the B-horror comedy *Bath Salt Zombies* (Dustin Mills 2013).
3. This is by no means to be an exhaustive informatic survey but certainly indicative and representative of a larger trend. Bibliometric analysis was conducted using the PubMed database on December 12, 2014.
4. See Canavan's chapter in this volume.
5. There are notable exceptions to the broad strokes outlined here that are based in medical/health humanities research, such as Shaka McGlotten and Lisa Jean Moore's (2013) use of the zombie as a framework through which to understand aging queer patients vis-à-vis the lure of revitalized sexual function through pharmacology.
6. Though in the section below I am mainly referring to macroparasites

(worms and plasmodia), there are notable examples of viruses that operate under similar pathogenic mechanism, such as the baculovirus that infects caterpillars and forces them to climb to the top of plants where they die and subsequently liquefy to propagate infection.

7. See also Webster and colleagues (2013). Once in the brain *T. gondii* interferes with neuroimmunological mechanisms to down-regulate immune response. This evasive adaption is similar to the cases were a porcine tapeworm makes it way to the brain of a human and forms a protective cyst to avoid immune response, also known as cysticercosis, a process that keeps both worm and host alive. If the parasite dies, the cyst dissolves and the immune system rushes to attack the foreign body, many times resulting in a potentially lethal inflammatory response (Meyer and Fried 2002, 32–25). *T. gondii* is also a feature in Mayra Grant's (2014) popular novel *Parasite*.
8. Google web search sorted by time, January 15, 2015.
9. See Smith's chapter in this volume for a theoretical deployment of Cazdyn's *Already Dead* with respect to the zombie.

10. A version of this comic can be accessed online at http://www.nationalgeographic .com/mindsuckers/rat.html.

REFERENCES

Adamo, Shelley A., and Joanne P. Webster. 2013. "Neural Parasitology: How Parasites Manipulate Host Behaviour." *Journal of Experimental Biology* 216 (1): 1–2.

Agamben, Giorgio. 1998. *Homo Sacer: Sovereign Power and Bare Life.* Translated by Daniel Heller-Roazen. Stanford, CA: Stanford University Press.

Boon, Kevin. 2011. "And the Dead Shall Rise." In *Better Off Dead: The Evolution of the Zombie as Post-Human*, edited by Deborah Christie and Sarah Juliet Lauro, 1–8. New York: Fordham University Press.

Brune, Jerome. 2013. "There Are Zombies among Us." *The Telegraph*, March 26. http://www.telegraph.co.uk/news/ science/9953571/There-are-zombies -among-us.html.

Burri, Regula Valérie, and Joseph Dumit. 2007. "Social Studies of Scientific Imaging and Visualization." In *The Handbook of Science and Technology Studies*, edited by Olga Amsterdamska, Edward J. Hackett, Michael E. Lynch, and Judy Wajcman, 297–317. Cambridge, MA: MIT Press.

Canavan, Gerry. 2010. "'We Are the Walking Dead': Race, Time, and Survival in Zombie Narrative." *Extrapolation* 51 (3): 431–53.

Cartwright, Lisa. 1995. *Screening the Body: Tracing Medicine's Visual Culture.* Minneapolis: University of Minnesota Press.

Cazdyn, Eric M. 2012. *The Already Dead: The New Time of Politics, Culture, and Illness.* Durham, NC: Duke University Press.

Clarke, Adele, Laura Mamo, Jennifer Ruth Fosket, Jennifer R. Fishman, and Janet K. Shim, eds. 2010. *Biomedicalization: Technoscience, Health, and Illness in the U.S.* Durham, NC: Duke University Press.

Cryan, J. F., and S. M. O'Mahony. 2011. "The Microbiome-Gut-Brain Axis: From Bowel to Behavior." *Neurogastroenterology and Motility* 23 (3): 187–92.

Czerwiec, MK, Michael Green, Ian Williams, Susan M. Squier, Kimberly Myers, and Scott Smith. 2015. *Graphic Medicine Manifesto.* University Park: Pennsylvania State University Press.

Daston, Lorraine, and Peter Galison. 2007. *Objectivity.* New York: Zone Books.

Davis, E. Wade. 1983. "The Ethnobiology of the Haitian Zombi." *Journal of Ethnopharmacology* 9 (1): 85–104.

Dumit, Joseph. 2004. *Picturing Personhood: Brain Scans and Biomedical Identity.* Princeton, NJ: Princeton University Press.

Eisner, Will. 2008. *Comics and Sequential Art: Principles and Practices from the Legendary Cartoonist.* New York: W. W. Norton.

Evans, Casey Dawn. 2009. "'They're Us': Infectious Trauma and the Zombie Apocalypse." PhD diss., University of Arkansas, 2009.

Fhlainn, Sorcha Ni. 2011. "All Dark Inside: De-humanization and Zombification in Postmodern Cinema." In *Better Off Dead: The Evolution of the Zombie as Post-Human*, edited by Deborah Christie and Sarah Juliet Lauro, 139–58. New York: Fordham University Press.

Flegr, Jaroslav. 2013. "Influence of Latent Toxoplasma Infection on Human Personality, Physiology and Morphology: Pros and Cons of the Toxoplasma-Human Model in Studying the Manipulation

Hypothesis." *Journal of Experimental Biology* 216 (1): 127–33.

Green, Michael J., and Kimberly R. Myers. 2010. "Graphic Medicine: Use of Comics in Medical Education and Patient Care." *BMJ: British Medical Journal (Overseas & Retired Doctors Edition)* 340 (7746): 574–77.

Hughes, David, Sandra Andersen, Nigel Hywel-Jones, Winanda Himaman, Johan Billen, and Jacobus Boomsma. 2011. "Behavioral Mechanisms and Morphological Symptoms of Zombie Ants Dying from Fungal Infection." *BMC Ecology* 11 (1): 13.

Khan, Ali S. 2011. "Preparedness 101: Zombie Apocalypse." *Centers for Disease Control and Prevention Public Health Matters Blog*, May 16. http://blogs.cdc .gov/publichealthmatters/2011/05/ preparedness-101-zombie-apocalypse/.

Kirkman, Robert, Tony Moore, and Charlie Adlard. 2003–. *The Walking Dead*. Comic book series. Berkeley, CA: Image Comics.

Lauro, Sarah Juliet, and Karen Embry. 2008. "A Zombie Manifesto: The Nonhuman Condition in the Era of Advanced Capitalism." *boundary 2* 35 (1): 85–108.

Mbembe, Achille. 2003. "Necropolitics." Translated by Libby Meintjes. *Public Culture* 15 (1): 11–40.

McCloud, Scott. 1994. *Understanding Comics: The Invisible Art*. New York: Harper Perennial.

McGlotten, Shaka, and Lisa Jean Moore. 2013. "The Geriatric Clinic: Dry and Limp: Aging Queers, Zombies, and Sexual Reanimation." *Journal of Medical Humanities* 34 (2): 261–68.

Meyer, D. A., and E. Fried. 2002. "Human Parasites and Surgical Intervention." In *Advances in Parasitology*, edited by John R. Baker, Ralph Muller, and David Rollinson. San Diego: Academic Press.

Ostherr, Kirsten. 2013. *Medical Visions: Producing the Patient through Film, Television, and Imaging Technologies*. Oxford, UK: Oxford University Press.

Seitz-Wald, Alex. 2013. "The Zombie Apocalypse That Wasn't: Bath Salts!" *Salon*, August 6. http://www.salon.com/2013/ 08/06/the_zombie_apocalypse_that _wasnt_bath_salts/.

Servitje, Lorenzo. 2015. "Keep Your Head in the Gutter: Engendering Empathy through Participatory Delusion in Christian de Metter's Graphic Adaptation of *Shutter Island*." *Journal of Medical Humanities* 36 (3): 1–18.

Silver, Maggie, James Archer, Bob Hobbs, Alissa Eckert, and Mark Conner. 2011. *Preparedness 101: Zombie Pandemic*. Atlanta: CDC / U.S. Department of Health and Human Services.

Squier, Susan. 2008. "So Long as They Grow Out of It: Comics, the Discourse of Developmental Normalcy, and Disability." *Journal of Medical Humanities* 29 (2): 71–88.

———. 2015. "The Use of Graphic Medicine for Engaged Scholarship." In *Graphic Medicine Manifesto*, by MK Czerwiec, Michael Green, Ian Williams, Susan M. Squier, Kimberly Myers, and Scott Smith, 41–65. University Park: Pennsylvania State University Press.

Squier, Susan, and J. Ryan Marks. 2014. "Introduction." *Configurations* 22 (2): 149–52.

Twombly, Matt. 2014. E-mail message to the author, December 30.

Wald, Priscilla. 2008. *Contagious: Cultures, Carriers, and the Outbreak Narrative*. Durham, NC: Duke University Press.

Webster, Joanne P., Maya Kaushik, Greg C. Bristow, and Glenn A. McConkey. 2013. "*Toxoplasma gondii* Infection, from Predation to Schizophrenia: Can Animal Behaviour Help Us Understand Human Behaviour?" *Journal of Experimental Biology* 216 (1): 99–112.

Weinersmith, Kelly, and Zen Faulkes. 2014. "Parasitic Manipulation of Hosts' Phenotype; or, How to Make a Zombie: An Introduction to the Symposium." *Integrative and Comparative Biology* 54 (2): 93–100.

Williams, Ian. 2012. "Graphic Medicine: Comics as Medical Narrative." *Medical Humanities* 38 (1): 21–27.

———. 2014. "Graphic Medicine." In *Medicine, Health, and the Arts: Approaches to the Medical Humanities*, edited by Victoria Bates, Alan Bleakley, and Sam Goodman, 64–84. London: Routledge.

———. 2015. "Comics and the Iconography of Illness." In *Graphic Medicine Manifesto*, by MK Czerwiec, Michael Green, Ian Williams, Susan M. Squier, Kimberly Myers, and Scott Smith, 143–64. University Park: Pennsylvania State University Press.

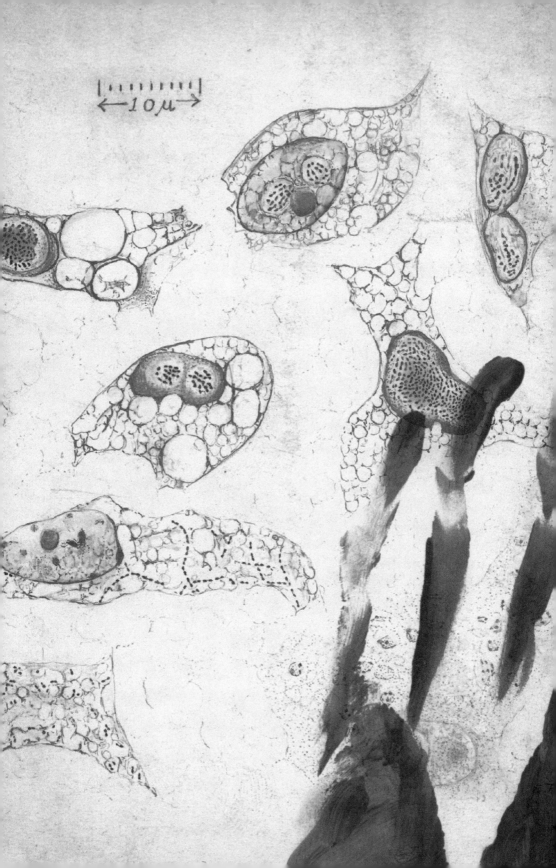

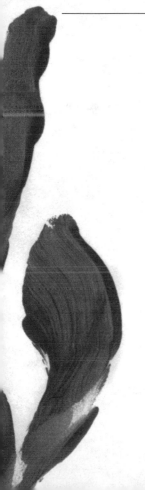

PART 1:
DIAGNOSING
ZOMBIE
CULTURE

1.

DON'T POINT THAT GUN AT MY MUM

Geriatric Zombies

Gerry Canavan

Academic analyses of zombie narratives have tended to read these stories as genocidal fantasies of unrestricted violence against monstrous Others with whom no sympathy is possible and who, as a result, can be murdered without guilt. The typical critical move, that is, has been to read such stories metaphorically, as murderous ideation against the raced, classed, and colonized subjects whose extermination is no longer wished for openly but whose difference is still perceived as a dire threat to white middle-class subjectivity in the industrialized West.[1] This is true even of more politically utopian readings of zombie narrative, such as Sarah Juliet Lauro and Karen Embry's widely cited "A Zombie Manifesto" (2008), which accedes to the basic terms of the violence but chooses instead to take the zombies' side, identifying their brutal destruction of the existing order as a sideways vision of a longed-for revolution. Novels, films, and video games may *nominally* be about fantastic encounters with zombies (or robots, or orcs, or alien invaders, or sentient apes), the argument goes, but on the more abstract level of ideology they are actually about reproducing and/or critically reexamining cultural narratives about who in real-world society is "killable" and who is not.

Without diminishing the importance of such readings, in this chapter I want to enrich this approach to zombie fantasy by introducing a new Other to the long list of politically sensitive topics that zombies can be seen to allegorize: the disabled or infirm body, particularly the elderly body. I argue that the zombie "resurgence" of the twenty-first century can and should be linked to the changing demographics of the industrialized world in that same period. After a decade languishing in low-budget, direct-to-video releases doomed to obscurity in the back rows of the video store, the zombie suddenly returns as an important mainstream cultural force in the 2000s precisely alongside the aging and decline of the World War II and boomer generations. To risk putting too fine a point on things, we have suddenly become acutely interested in slow-moving, degenerating bodies and forgetful minds with violently altered personalities at the very moment that cultural concern over the progressive and degenerative conditions that strike the elderly (such as Alzheimer's, post-stroke symptomology, advanced cancers, aphasias, multiple sclerosis, Huntington's and Parkinson's diseases, and the like) is at an all-time high. Likewise, these ravenous undead figures have become important cultural markers at the very moment that anxiety about the ability of younger and poorer generational cohorts to support the swelling ranks of the elderly over the coming decades has become a potent force in Western politics. Thus we frequently see in recent zombie fantasies (and in related fantasies of decrepit immortals who refuse to die, such as José Saramago's [2008] novel *Death with Interruptions* or the UK television series *Torchwood*'s fourth-season arc, *Miracle Day* [2011]) the repressed expression of a real and increasingly urgent *intergenerational* struggle—one that is complicated by the unhappy realization that *this* sort of "zombiism" is in fact the universal fate of anyone sufficiently "lucky" to live long enough to experience the inevitable breakdown of their mind and body.

In this chapter I trace the zombie's allegorization of aging and senescence through a number of the zombie texts that have emerged since the explosive popularity of Danny Boyle's film *28 Days Later* (2003) and Robert Kirkman's *The Walking Dead* (comic 2003–; television 2010–; video game 2012–). But my focus will be on my identification of a newer, smaller subgenre of zombie texts that has risen to prominence only recently, in which the zombie's original subjectivity is mostly or entirely retained, and they are even able to talk in complete and complex sentences. The novel assertion that zombies might remember, speak, and feel—albeit in ways that parallel the cognitive and emotional disabilities associated with old age—interrupts the logic of radical inhumanity that had previously licensed unrestricted violence against them, recasting the zombie not as the monster that can only be killed but as the transformed loved one who must somehow still be cared for, despite their unhappy metamorphosis. It is in these newer texts (which have frequently originated in the medium of comics) that the implicit connection between zombie fantasy, disability, and gerontology I am uncovering becomes most visible to us; the physical and mental anguish that the zombies experience in "talking zombie" narratives maps directly on to the suffering that is inherent in growing old—which the zombies' new ability to speak allows them to communicate to the people that had once been (and, sometimes, may still be) both their victims and their killers.

Planet of Zombies

The industrialized world is growing older. Japan faces steeply declining birth rates at the same moment as a rapidly aging population remains; these trends have only accelerated since the 1990s, with record population decline in 2014. The birth rate in Japan is only 1.39 per woman, well under replacement rate, while 20 percent of the population is over the age of sixty-five; by one estimate, in 2060 the country's population will have shrunk by nearly a third (to 87 million, from 127 million today), with 40 percent of that population over sixty-five (Panda 2014). And Japan, while an extreme case, is by no means unique; the combination of declining birth rates with a graying population exists across the globe. The birth rate in many countries in Europe has dipped below replacement rate as well; as of 2004 the birth rate was approximately 1.5 per woman across the EU, and as low as 1.3 in Germany, Spain, and Italy (see "Old Europe" 2004). The United States has remained above replacement rate largely due to the effects of immigration, though this has produced its own demographic panic in an aging white majority anticipating its own imminent transition to "majority minority" status (which has in turn produced fearful popular rhetoric about uncontrollable zombic "hordes" crossing the border). Still, the projections of a graying America suggest that a huge transformation of the country's demographics will be underway over the coming decades; in 2014 the Census Bureau projected that 84 million Americans will be sixty-five or older by 2050, more than 20 percent of the population, compared to fewer than 10 percent in 1970 (Williams 2014).

Although many of the effects of these demographic changes have not yet been felt with great intensity, sharp increases in healthcare spending and the growing need for pension expenditures (both public and private) have already been an important economic force across the 2000s—as have high-profile attempts (in Detroit and elsewhere) to renege on those pension obligations in the name of other budgetary priorities, notably debt repayment and cost-shifting. Just as important is the anticipation of the more radical changes that, we are told, will soon be necessary as a result of anticipated trends. Al Gore's famous "Social Security lockbox" from the 2000 US presidential campaign was only the opening salvo of fifteen years of debt- and deficit-related anxiety in American politics, much of it addressed to graying, increasingly conservative baby boomers worried about both the future "we" will be leaving for "our children," as well as their own ability to survive in the new world of austerity projected to be right around the corner. This vision of austerity is so robust as to perversely transform even longer life expectancy—that most hallowed marker of human achievement—into a pessimistic economic indicator, at least within the pages of the *Wall Street Journal*: "Good news for Americans: You are living longer. The bad news: The longer life span doesn't bode well for the corporate pension plans that are supposed to support workers into old age" (Fitzpatrick 2014). The long, scorched-earth policy fight over 2009's Affordable Care Act, popularly known as Obamacare, is only the most obvious example of this wide- ranging and widely felt civic crisis. To the Democratic left Obamacare signifies an attempt to "bend" the curve of healthcare costs as they are projected to continue to spike as a result of new treatments and an aging population, while to the Republican right Obamacare signals the emergence of "death panels" that will determine which lives have now become too costly to sustain—a list that members of the aging white male demographic of Fox News and the *Wall Street Journal* feel certain will target them, first and foremost.

These public policy shifts are mirrored by changes on the personal level of the home or the family. The first baby boomers turned fifty in 1996 and reached the traditional US retirement age (sixty-five) in 2011; the youngest baby boomers turned fifty in 2015. The largest demographic cohort in Amer- ican history is thus now encountering the diseases and conditions associated with aging that their own parents suffered and died from a generation pre- viously (or in many cases are *still* suffering from): slowdowns in speed and agility; senility and dementia; cancers; diabetes; strokes; progressive and degenerative conditions like Parkinson's, Huntington's, multiple sclerosis, Alzheimer's, and so on. Many of these conditions are associated with per- sonality changes, sometimes causing disturbing, bizarre, or violent behav- ior—while others are associated with a new condition of physical weakness or with severe depression, senility, or delusions. The family memory of the decline and death of parents—needless to say, often quite traumatic regard- less of the cause—and the anticipation of one's own imminent decline to come has led to these kinds of conditions having new visibility in American culture, both parents struggling with their own aging and for adult children wondering how to care for their declining parents.

The general stress of aging, and the stress of caring for aging parents, has been an important subject of popular attention across the 2000s, in every register: political, medicinal, ethical, economic, religious. *The Notebook* (Nick Cassavetes 2004) may be the most prominent recent film to feature characters with Alzheimer's disease and their caretakers, but the condition has been featured in a host of other well-received films in and outside the United States (perhaps most notably *Away from Her* [Sarah Polley 2006] and *Still Alice* [Richard Glatzer and Wash Westmoreland 2014]) as well as on television in *Grey's Anatomy*, *Raising Hope*, and even the surrealist cartoon *Adventure Time*. I choose Alzheimer's as my example here precisely because, as Susan M. Behuniak (2011, 77–78) among others has demonstrated, the particular symptomology of Alzheimer's has very frequently led comment-ers to compare it to "living death," and Alzheimer's patients to zombies themselves:

> Seven characteristics are associated with zombies by Romero's trope: exceptional physical characteristics, lack of self-recognition, failure to recognise others, cannibalisation of living human beings, the exponential spreading of this plague, the resulting horror of those still unafflicted, and the zombie's overwhelming hopelessness that makes death a preferred alternative than continued existence. . . .
>
> Three aspects of the zombie trope—appearance, loss of self, and loss of the ability to recognise others—have been directly applied to people with AD. Three other aspects—the epidemic threat, wide-spread cultural terror, and death as preferable to becoming an animated corpse—are referenced by way of implication in describ-ing the disease itself. The remaining aspect of the zombie trope—cannibalism—is applied both to patients and to the affect their disease has on others.

The "stigma" resulting from this metaphorical slippage between the fantastic condition and real-world medicine, Behuniak argues, "is powerful enough to replace compassion with fear, hope with despair, and empathy with dis-gust" (77). Carmelo Aquilina and Julian C. Hughes (2006, 143) have similarly suggested that the allegorical link between zombiism and old age has con-tributed to a culture in which "people with dementia can be treated as already dead and as walking corpses to be both pitied and feared, despite their obvious signs of life." Elizabeth Herskovits (1995, 153) has even gone so far as to claim that the popular conception of Alzheimer's—and perhaps the diagnosis as such—is, in itself, a "monsterizing of senility." And this is only one very prominent condition; we might easily make similar lists associated with Huntington's disease, multiple sclerosis, Parkinson's disease, cancers, strokes, diabetes, or any other number of conditions that strike in or after late middle age, each with their own set of "zombic" symptoms that can be used to differentiate them from the normative ideal of the nondisabled body.

In accordance with this line of thinking, it is my suggestion in this chapter that this cultural milieu—changing bodies, and their changing minds, and the difficult forging of new relationships between loved ones that are made necessary by these changes—is as important an etiology for the renewed interest in the zombie following the release of *28 Days Later* in 2003 as were the events of 9/11 and the war on terror to which such texts have usually been related.[2] Much of the beginning of *28 Days Later*—before the zombies emerge—registers an anxiety that is easily linked to family, especially to parents and the threats they can pose to children. Very early in the film, a long shot on a wall memorializing the dead lingers on a child's drawing of his or her parents, with the "Daddy" clearly wielding a knife and threatening the others. Shortly thereafter the protagonist, Jim (Cillian Murphy), first encounters the infected in a church; the first words Jim speaks in the film after the lengthy silent opening are "Hello? Hello? Father?" to a priest whom he must then hit over the head. Jim then goes to his parents' house, only to see they have killed themselves during the outbreak. Later, one of the most vivid and disturbing scenes in the film occurs when Frank (Brendan Gleeson) becomes infected with the "rage virus" and, out of nowhere, suddenly attacks the group, including his terrified daughter, Hannah (Megan Burns)—in one terrible instant transforming him from the loving father he had always been to a brutal attacker.

This theme of zombic family—or, more precisely, a zombiism that interrupts the circuit of family—is echoed and extended by an important scene in the zombie comedy *Shaun of the Dead* (Edgar Wright 2004), from which this chapter draws its title. When Shaun (Simon Pegg)'s mother is infected by the zombie virus, the entire tone of the film suddenly changes; what had previously been a comedic "romp" through an apocalyptic London becomes instead an unexpectedly sad rumination on the loss of one's parent. Shaun, who has previously killed zombies without remorse, cannot allow his mother to experience the same fate; against the members of his group who insist that she, too, must be put down, he screams, "Don't point that gun at my mum!" In this moment of rupture, the very telos of zombie narrative is temporarily suspended by the power of Shaun's love for his mother—though, in the end, Shaun must give in to inevitability and is forced to shoot her after all.

The first issue of Robert Kirkman's long-running comic book series *The Walking Dead*, like *28 Days Later*, also begins with its protagonist, Rick Grimes, waking up from a coma in an abandoned hospital. The series, like *28 Days Later* and *Shaun of the Dead*, is similarly constructed around a logic of shattered domesticity, with characters frequently losing (or forced to murder) either biological or ersatz family members. But the mood of *The Walking Dead* is made much darker than either *28 Days Later* or *Shaun of the Dead* by two significant structural changes. First, there is simply its open-ended nature; Kirkman has often said his ambition is to write a zombie movie that never ends, that piles on the horrors issue after issue after issue forever.[3] But second and more crucially there is his shift away from the logic of outbreak and infection back toward something closer to the metaphysical or existential nightmare that drove George Romero's original *Night of the Living Dead* (1968). Rather than a contagion, Kirkman's zombies are an ontology; in the universe of *The Walking Dead*, *everyone* is "infected." Everyone reanimates as a zombie shortly after they die, with catastrophic damage to the head either pre- or postmortem being the only possible way to prevent this dreaded fate. This leads to Rick's well-known rant, early in the comic series, that explains the buried pun in the series title: "You people don't know what we are! We're surrounded by the DEAD. We're among them—and when we finally give up we become them! We're living on borrowed time here. Every minute of our life is a minute we steal from them! You see them out there. You KNOW that when we die—we become them. You think we hide behind walls to protect us from the walking dead? Don't you get it? We ARE the walking dead! WE are the walking dead" (issue 24, pp. 19–22). The splash page's close-up on Rick's battered, bloodied face—wrapped in bandages from a severe head injury—is testament to how thin a line separates "them" from "us." We could any of us cross over at any moment.

In *"We're All Infected": Essays on AMC's "The Walking Dead" and the Fate of the Human*, a recent essay collection concerning the television adaptation of the comic series, the imminence of this change is linked to the thin line separating nondisabled persons from their potential future as disabled subjects. Several of the book's contributors tease out important links between the Romero/Kirkman-style zombie and the larger ideology of medicine, particularly with respect to the elderly. Xavier Aldana Reyes (2014, 148), for instance, focuses on what he calls the "dying undead" to call new attention to the fact that the comic's Walkers (i.e., zombies) are slowly "ceasing to exist through gradual erosion and physical decay"; while the Walkers themselves are "oblivious" to this fact, "the series takes great pains . . . to make a point of their suffering." Gary Farnell (2014, 178) takes up the *Walking Dead* zombie as a medicalized and disabled subject through explanation of one particular condition we have already noted as being linked to aging and senility, aphasia, the loss of either written or spoken language; one subhead asks, "What If Zombies Could Talk as Well as Walk?" But it is only Dave Beisecker (2014, 178), in the final pages of the book's afterword, who makes what is the final and necessary allegorical leap:

> Let us suppose that the zombies are an allegory for an aging "baby boomer" demographic. After all, in their ceaseless wandering and bewildered expressions, zombies can bear a striking resemblance to those afflicted by Alzheimer's, which has been called the defining affliction (and perhaps greatest fear) of the baby-boom generation. Indeed, the comparison seems apt. Every day, over 10,000 baby-boomers inexorably "crossover" into retirement age, and the overwhelming weight of their numbers, especially by comparison to subsequent "Generations X and Y," threatens to bring down our health care system and social security net (or so we are told).

Rereading the zombie as a figure for the elderly transforms our attitude toward the zombie, giving new energy to possibilities condemned in the larger series like (to note Beisecker's examples) Morgan's inability to kill his zombified wife, or Hershel's locking his deceased family and neighbors in his barn pending treatment. If zombies are simply another stage of human life, the firm line that separates "us" from "them" (and makes "us" worthy of protection while "them" worthy only of extermination) becomes erased, impossible to see. "If aging is the affliction," Beisecker goes on, "*we are all infected*. . . . In the natural course of things, there might come an awkward time of twilight in which we are neither ourselves, nor are we dead" (212–13).

This critical intervention necessarily pushes us away from the eliminationist logic that governs most zombie narratives toward an ethical paradigm more conducive to the field of medicine than war. Instead of wild animals being put down, such zombies look more like patients (perhaps our own parents) being euthanized—or even, unthinkably, *not being killed at all*, but rather treated and cared for. At the same time, this alternative way of thinking about zombies directs us toward the zombic body as a genuine problem for the medical field, outside the fantasy: what do we *do* with bodies whose intensity of suffering, or extreme cognitive decline, or total non-responsiveness, seem to have pushed them outside the realm of human life into some other category altogether? Even texts that flirt with a medicinal context, like *Torchwood: Miracle Day*, often collapse back into eliminationist thinking as hospitals begin to run short on beds, doctors become overwhelmed by their patients, and unpaid bills begin to pile up. Such thinking dialectically loops us back to the intergenerational anxiety with which I began this section: the fear of a coming planet of zombies, filled with decaying bodies that can no longer do productive work but which cannot be disposed of either. How do we break out of this trap? Is another zombie possible?

Can the Zombie Speak?

At the start of the 2000s, zombies were seen as a niche interest at best; when Robert Kirkman sold *The Walking Dead* to Image Comics, for instance, he was allowed to use zombies only on the promise that "the zombies were actually animated by an alien race that was preparing to invade Earth by disrupting its infrastructure"; the idea of a "zombie comic" seemed that bizarre and that unworkable from a financial perspective (Johnston 2012).[4] More than a decade into *The Walking Dead*, now zombie comics are everywhere, a staple of the industry—and they have become quite diverse, even sometimes taking up possibilities for zombie narrative that move beyond the usual forced logic of crisis and extermination. One such narrative possibility that has become popular in the intervening years is the psychic repudiation of the logic that drove the death of Shaun's mother: what if Shaun's mother *did not* have to die? Even *Shaun of the Dead* itself took up this possibility as its closing joke; at the end of the film Shaun's infected friend, Ed (Nick Frost), is kept locked in a shed in the backyard rather than killed, where the two can play video games together. But in a new subgenre of zombie fantasy this possibility of rapprochement with the zombie takes center stage, facilitated by an important shift in the zombie mythos: the new ability of zombies to think, feel, and speak.

In *Warm Bodies* (novel 2010; film 2013), originally based on a short story called "I Am a Zombie Filled with Love," the unthinking and lumbering zombie is revealed to retain some type of human interiority, in a kind of fantastic Locked-in Syndrome—which in the fairy-tale logic of the narrative is able to be unlocked, and reversed, with a kiss. Other recent filmic and televisual treatments extend this shift to its natural endpoint, imagining zombies as fully articulate subjects simply suffering from a highly unusual medical ailment.[5] These texts implicitly and often explicitly take up the idea of zombiism as a kind of disability, an ongoing condition that can (at least potentially) be managed through love and care. The title of Margaret Atwood and Naomi Alderman's recent novella *The Happy Zombie Sunrise Home*, first published on Wattpad.com, is perhaps illustrative here. Rather than the locked-down hospital of *28 Days Later* and *The Walking Dead*, the militarized inner city of *World War Z* (novel 2006; film 2013) or Colson Whitehead's *Zone One* (2011), the juvenile detention center of M. R. Carey's *The Girl with All the Gifts* (2014), or the death camps of *Torchwood: Miracle Day*, Atwood and Alderman's surprisingly sweet mother-daughter story imagines the zombie as more properly inhabiting something like a nursing home.

Of course, the mere innovation of talking zombies, by itself, does not necessarily promote sympathy or an ethics of care. Warren Ellis's comic *Blackgas* (2007, with Max Fiumara and Ryan Waterhouse), for instance, would seem to contain all the elements that might provoke a zombie ethics alternative to the need for killing, but there is ultimately no change in its narrative trajectory. The zombie outbreak happens during a visit to one protagonist's childhood home; after a chase during the initial outbreak, the characters encounter Tyler's mother in this psychologically crucial space. The panels are drawn to evoke the way horror films delay the reveal of their creature, with Tyler's mother's face first shrouded in shadow, then obscured by shots of the sides and back of her head. Tyler's mother at first says she is OK but is quickly revealed to be carrying the head of Tyler's father, his dismembered penis stuffed into his mouth. She has been changed by exposure to the black gas, though there is an implication that these changes reflect an extreme loosening of inhibitions rather than a genuinely radical transformation of the self: "Had enough of his shit. All his shit. . . . All the things I always thought about doing. I just did them. So hungry now." Finally, we see the monster dead-on (part 2).[6] Her unkempt, filthy appearance and flat affect reinforce the sense of psychological break suggested by her newfound hostility, even hatefulness—all personality changes associated with dementia, senility, and adult-onset neurodegenerative disease. This horrifying encounter with the mother does not produce any significant sympathy in the characters, however; she is quickly dispatched, with Tyler left to wonder only whether he had told his parents he loved them when he last saw them, as the zombie narrative continues down its well-trod, gory path.

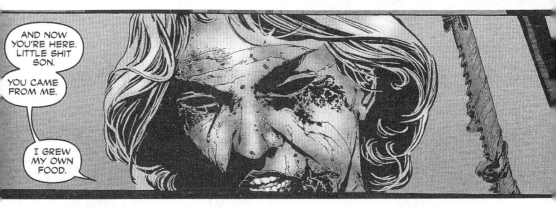

1.1 From *Blackgas* by Warren Ellis and Max Fiumara. Reprinted by permission of Avatar Press.

The zombies in the DC Comics (2009–10) crossover event *Blackest Night* evokes a similar relationship to family: they are the corpses of fallen heroes reanimated by the "Black Lantern" power of the villainous Nekron and able to speak. In the context of DC's system of "legacy" heroes, this entails an intense focus on literal parents as well as mentors and father figures, alongside spouses and comrades. Here, as in *Blackgas*, the presentation is something more akin to demon possession than mere aging; what these lost fathers, mothers, and mentors say is always wicked and always hurtful, with none of the original heroism and self-sacrifice that had marked their earlier appearances as living heroes—and usually augmented by a disturbing and out-of-character sexual aggressivity that constitutes a key locus of horror in the comic. Needless to say, there are any number of late-adulthood conditions that mirror this sort of disturbing and dramatic personality shift, though as with Behuniak's discussion of Alzheimer's or the earlier discussion of *The Walking Dead* what is at work here is not so much a one-to-one presentation of specific symptoms as the "cumulative stock image . . . [forming] a powerful metaphor that is utterly recognizable and so familiar that only a few need to be invoked to imply the others" (Behuniak 2011, 78). Here the Black Lanterns' zombic presentation as decrepit, nasty walking corpses evokes a hostility to infirm bodies and non-neurotypical minds that draws on ageist and ableist assumptions about what is "normal" to generate the sense of revolting abjection on which the story hinges—without ever directly naming any one particular condition as the object of the allegory. What is built out of these kinds of zombie stories is really something more like a mood than a metaphor: the general sense that the older generation is, or at any moment could turn into, a sinister and threatening horror, a crisis, a problem to be "solved."

The story's science fantasy—that this is all the unnatural work of a strange alien technology—provides the cognitive buffer that flattens and legitimates this antagonism: the Black Lanterns may have the bodies of loved ones, and may know the things they know, but they are nonetheless onto-logically distinct, and so the series as a whole is able to replicate the familiar exterminative logic of typical zombie narratives without complication. It is only in the spinoff series *Blackest Night: The Flash* that the psychic closeness of these zombies to the deceased loved ones *does* begin to intrude on the need to eliminate the monsters without compunction; the second Captain Boomerang chooses to side with the monstrous Black Lantern corpse of his father (the first Boomerang) over the combined team of heroes, antiheroes, and villains that is fighting zombies in Central City. "I can't let you hurt my father," he says to his compatriots. "Don't be stupid, kid. That's not your father. It's a walking bag of bones," replies Captain Cold. But Boomerang is defiant: "I'm going to help you, Dad," he says to the zombie. "I know how to bring you back" (Johns and Ries 2008, issue 2, last page). For his part, the zombie recognizes his son immediately: "Owen? Son?" In the panel, Boo-merang I does not even look that monstrous—nor, indeed, all that different from the nearby Captain Cold, who is calling for Boomerang I's immediate execution.

As the narrative progresses, Boomerang II even brings living people to feed to the zombie, in a mistaken belief that this will help revivify his lost father; his karmic punishment for this bizarre mix of love and sociopathy is to be fed to his father himself in due course (Johns and Ries 2008, issue 3).[7] Weirdly, though, Boomerang II's gambit to save his father does ultimately pay off, albeit in a way he never expected. A small number of the Black Lanterns (including Boomerang I) *are* magically revivified as part of the outcome of the story and returned to their old lives, with their original personalities and restored health—hopelessly blurring the supposedly clear ontological distinction between these creatures' "normal" living state and their corpses' status as demonic Black Lanterns.

Other comic treatments land still elsewhere on the continuum between monstrosity and sympathy. In Marvel's *Marvel Zombies* (2005–6), written by *The Walking Dead*'s Robert Kirkman, it is again the heroes who have become zombified, despondently consuming every other living thing on the planet (and the galaxy, and the universe, and the next universe over . . .) in their endless search for food. Although the Marvel universe's various genius-level intellects have been affected, no cure is available to them; as they begin to lose their cognitive abilities and forget their lives[8] the zombies can only reflect dyspeptically on their situation as they degrade both mentally and physically. But unlike DC's storyline, the Marvel zombies have not been turned into killers and perverts; they behave this way only when they are hungry. Instead of psychological discomfort, the artistic focus is instead on body horror: multiple characters lose limbs, Captain America is missing most of his skull, and the Wasp is reduced to just a ghastly head. Their moods swing wildly from rage to mad hunger to suicidal regret, though nothing gives the heroes hope. "I don't want to figure anything out!" screams Spider-Man, thinking of how he ate both his wife, Mary Jane Watson, and his beloved Aunt May. "I think I just want to die!" (Kirkman and Phillips 2005, part 1).

As with the DC Comics event, the sheer *oldness* of the heroes itself helps to fuel the symbolic link to actual old age: these are characters that were invented as teenagers in the 1960s or even the 1940s but who have never really aged, characters for whom the normal passage of time has somehow been suspended altogether. These characters should be ancient; by now they *should* all be retired, or in nursing homes, or dead. Transforming Iron Man and Captain America into zombies is in some sense no transformation at all, so much as a revealing of what these out-of-time characters have been for decades as they have become totally divorced from the mid-century cultural context from which they (and the baby boomers more generally) sprang.[9] Whereas DC's *Blackest Night* ends with a fantasy of resurrection and revivification for its moribund characters, returning them to their lost and longed for state of vibrant youth, Marvel's more cynical zombie narrative embraces this state of furious obsolescence. In this story the zombies are triumphant, taking over the planet-devouring alien Galactus to threaten the rest of their universe, and ultimately the entire multiverse, with their bottomless resentment for those who are still alive.

Marvel's *Night of the Living Deadpool* (2014) achieves a similar effect of temporal disjunction in a different way: the book is drawn in black and white, evoking the film stock of its cinema namesake; only Deadpool himself appears in color, as if he is wandering around within the frame of the old movie. *Night of the Living Deadpool* amplifies the regret and angst found in the zombies of *Marvel Zombies*: the infected are likewise driven to horrific violence they would have never contemplated in their previous lives. Here, though, rather than simply succumbing to their uncanny hunger, they are constantly *aware* of this difference, utterly horrified by it and unable to explain to themselves what they are doing or to find the capacity to stop. "Don't *want* to do this . . . can't . . . stop myself," mutters the miserable zombie that Deadpool encounters near the beginning of the book; "Oh, this is awful." The violence against the zombies that appears in the story accordingly shifts from gleeful extermination to something more like euthanasia or mercy killing. It is mournful, and miserable, rather than exhilarating. "Please . . . please . . . kill me," the zombie begs. Deadpool does so, only to be quickly confronted (in a long panel that runs horizontally across two pages) by a throng of zombies, all speaking over one another, begging for death: "So sorry"; "Don't let me . . ."; "Someone find my daughter"; "Please help"; "I had a good life"; "Kill me next." Here it is the confusion of neurodegeneration that reigns supreme in zombification, the loss of self-identity that comes with loss of control. These zombies are not inhuman, or nonpersons; they are *suffering*. Deadpool—a character whose narration frequently bounces off the fourth wall—is frustrated by this violation of the implied contract of zombie narrative. He has been cheated: "I've played video games! Whacking dead folks is supposed to be fun!" (Bunn and Rosanas 2014, issue 1).

Zombie Families/Zombie Love

Other "talking zombie" texts, outside the superhero genre, push us still further from the routinized logic of violent and relentless extermination toward an alternative mode of thinking about zombic bodies. Tim Seeley and Mike Norton's *Revival* (2012–), a "rural noir," is set in an isolated town in Wisconsin where the dead have risen. The "Revivers" in the small town of Wausau need to reintegrate into their lives in a town that now faces quarantine from a panicked nation around it; the protagonist, Dana, is the police detective put in charge of "the Revitalized Citizen Arbitration Team," a special task force devoted to crimes involving the Revivers. "I've spent the last few weeks interviewing all the Revivers," her father, the local police chief, tells her. "Most of them, they're just like they used to be. But some of them . . . Anyway, your first case came in the morning." That is to say, some of them are different, in ways that are genuinely frightening—but not *all* of them (vol. 1).

That first case involves an older woman (naturally, a Reviver) who keeps regrowing her teeth and then pulling them out with pliers so she can fit in her dentures; by the end of the issue she has brutally murdered her daughter, screaming incoherently that Dana made her do it. The page uses the same horror-movie strategy as *Blackgas* to obscure a full view of the zombie before its reveal—but this time the depiction is not that of an eyeless monster, but simply the face of an old, frightened woman who does not understand what is happening to her, or even the monstrous thing she is about to do. The comic continues: "Heaven wouldn't take me. Made me stay in Purgatory. . . . Just wanted to rest. Wanted to sit at the side of the Lord. I was going to sing with the angels . . . Everyone thinks it's a miracle, but then they whisper and point. Ask me to heal them." The same woman revives again and escapes the morgue, arriving at her daughter's funeral to ask, unknowing, "Oh, honey, who did this to you?" before transforming into a more traditionally mindless zombie and attacking the stunned onlookers (vol. 1).

Another Reviver, an elderly man, seems to have come back to a kind of catatonic senility. But those around him think he's faking. "You think he's just some poor old man drooling and shitting his pants," his son-in-law says during a guns-drawn confrontation with Dana. "But he's not. He's faking it. He's one of *them*. He died, and he came back. And, he's . . . he's got something wrong in that brain. He's sick and he's fucking evil." And the son-in-law is more or less right. Anders *is* faking it, as he seeks revenge on the daughter who murdered him with the help of her adulterous lover, her own stepbrother, for their inheritance: "You'd already lived, Daddy. So well . . . So

1.2 From *Revival*, volume 1, *You're among Friends*, by Tim Seeley and Mike Norton. Reprinted by permission of Image Comics.

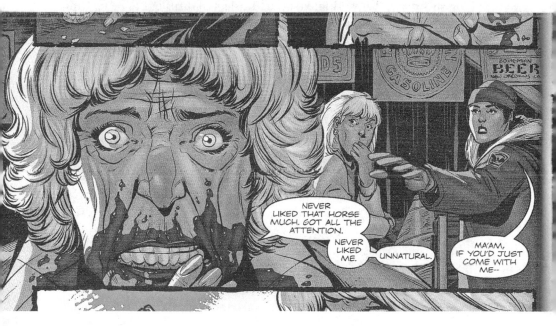

l-long. But our lives couldn't even get started." Anders does murder her, though he takes little joy in it, and pointedly asks Dana a question that we can now recognize as being at the center of twenty-first-century zombie fiction: "How will the next generation thrive . . . if the old generation doesn't die?" (vol. 2).

Other Revivers experience similar breakdowns, not all of them murderous: some experience severe health problems (or repeated deaths), or losses of affect, or fugue states. Not all—seemingly not even most—are murderous, though the narrative seems to hint that violent and psychotic outbursts may be associated with Revival on some level. But the narrative never endorses the attitude that the appropriate "answer" to this problem could be to round up the Revivers and murder or imprison them all, any more than such a thing could be suggested about the mentally ill or the elderly in a real-world context; whenever such an idea is posited, it is revealed to be monstrous and roundly rejected by the more sympathetic characters. Even the reliance on the fantasy of a noble small-town police department—run by a father-daughter team—points toward the notions of family and community that ground the series. Tellingly, it is almost always outsiders to the community who suggest these extreme measures, and characters within the community who resist them. Instead of elimination, the Revivers indicate a difficult population that must be carefully managed, with care and love, rather than with exterminative violence. When it is revealed that there actually is something supernatural at work in Wausau, the demon turns out to be hunting *Revivers*, who need to be protected from *it*. Similarly, many of the "cases" Dana encounters are actually about those who would seek to exploit Revivers—those who, for instance, would try to transport their body parts for sale as an aphrodisiac or exotic food, outside the quarantine zone—rather than the Revivers themselves as a threat. Most Revivers, even while experiencing disturbing personality changes, remain cherished and loved, like Dana's own sister; others are children, whose periodic odd or disturbing behavior does not push them outside the boundaries of love and protection, or our sympathy, or of the human. (When one terrified Reviver child *is* abandoned by her parents and institutionalized in volume 3, our sympathies are overwhelmingly with the child.) Even a second confrontation with Anders sees him framed as someone who "got a second chance" but "blew it by being a piece of shit" (vol. 4)—suggesting that other Revivers could choose to embrace their better selves instead. Frequently, Dana and others need to intervene to prevent the Revivers from hurting themselves, either out of guilt or out of a misplaced sense that their loved ones would be better off without them. When Diane, the Revived wife of Ken Dillisch, the town's mayor, tries to harm herself, his answer is clear: "Now you see, right? Why I can't let them take the Revivers away? Why they can't put them in some lab or a camp? . . . She's my wife. I'm not letting someone else tell me what's best for her. And I'm sure as shit not letting some fucking towelhead from the CDC cut her up. I just need her to remember that she has so much to live for, even more now" (vol. 4).[10] Of course his methods of dealing with her are also deeply inappropriate—he ties her up and confines her in a misguided (and ultimately failed) effort to protect her from herself. Both husband and wife would undoubtedly benefit from responsible medical intervention (as opposed to police/military violence) aimed at caring for their needs and alleviating their suffering. The Revival crisis calls for doctors and psychologists—care teams, not soldiers.

Even these terms get muddied as the series progresses; at the end of volume 5, *Gathering of Waters* (collecting issues 24–29), we see the mayor's wife set off a suicide bomb at a press conference that outed her as a Reviver, killing dozens including her husband, while in issue 31 and onward it is revealed that the monster apparently hunting Revivers is a being of intense *love* as well as horrific violence. Despite the language of sympathy and care that is used by outsiders, in bad faith, to justify locking more and more Revivers away, the audience is meant to recoil from this logic of instrumentalization and institutionalization (which here is nothing but extermination by another name). "The ultimate horror in science fiction," Carlos Clarens (1997, 134) has written, "is neither death nor destruction but dehumanization." Accordingly the overarching ethos of *Revival* is the rejection of zombie narrative's familiar logic of dehumanization, and an insistence instead that the bounds of love, community, and family must somehow be stronger than the uncanny strangeness of Revival, even when this seems hardest to imagine.

At the furthest end of the spectrum from the extermination of *Blackgas* and *Blackest Night* we find Matthew Shepherd and Roy Boney, Jr.'s *Dead Eyes Open* (2005), which abolishes any need for zombie extermination entirely. Echoing the identity politics and self discovery discourse of *In the Flesh*, here zombiism is presented as just another chronic health condition in a world already full of them. Dr. John Requin, the psychiatrist at the story's center, is living a lie when the book begins: he is actually a zombie, and he worries his patients are beginning to catch on. His daughter fears, despite her mother and father's assurances to the contrary, that he might try to "eat her brains"; in fact, his condition simply requires a diet high in protein, mostly tofu, and keeping the house a little cooler than the living find comfortable. But still, he is lethargic and emits an unusual smell. "I suffer from a strange affliction," John soon announces at a press conference, when he is forced out of the metaphorical closet to lead a Cabinet-level task force dedicated to "Returner Affairs"—"but I am still fundamentally the same person I have always been" (chap. 2).

His role as the first liaison of Returner Affairs is hardly easy. The federal government had been covertly killing Returners whenever they were discovered, in an effort to keep the truth under wraps—but the rate of Return has gone from one in a million to one in six hundred and the secret is now far too big to contain. Some of the zombies are criminals or terrorists—usually in violent counterreaction to the government's own exterminative bent—but most are simply normal people trying to return to their lives in peace. Returners are simply a new situation that must be confronted not with "fear or superstition" but with reason and empathy. "Research is being conducted," John promises. "We will understand this phenomenon . . . and we will get through it together" (chap. 2).

The world will simply need to change, to find some way to adapt to a new class of "Humans Plus"[11] who barely eat, never get sick, and have no need to sleep. We see glimpses of the changing economic and legal context throughout the story, especially around the new practice of willing one's money to oneself: as one Returner puts it, "Money's not an issue with me, gentlemen. When I died, I was richer than Croesus. And I'm not getting any poorer. Do you know how many retirees are leaving their money to themselves? We don't need medical, nursing, special care. Money's not the issue" (chap. 6). The threat here, as in *Revival*, is in some ways the inverse to the threat of aging focused on earlier in this chapter—we are worried not that the older generation might die but that they might *never* die, hoarding and consuming necessary resources even as they persist as shadows of themselves. At the same time *Dead Eyes Open* also reverses the zombie body as an object of horror to turn it into an object of utopian fantasy: now it is the fantasy of a body that (at least potentially) might magically de-age, or might never get old at all. This is in fact what motivates the story's final antagonist, the murderous general, in his plan for Returner genocide: "Think, John. Undying billionaires in Arctic mansions, issuing orders to every continent. Returner soldiers fighting wars that never end. Media dominated by people that never eat, never get sick. A dead world." But John looks to the future, suggesting that the zombie condition may not be something monstrous or unnatural but instead (echoing a common euphemism

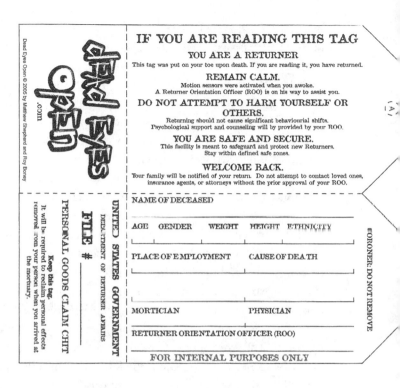

1.3 From *Dead Eyes Open* by Matthew Shepherd and Roy Boney, Jr. Reprinted by permission of the artists.

for aging) "just another phase of life" to which we all must find ways to adapt (chap. 6).

Dead Eyes Open deploys a number of the tropes common to the "zombie extermination" version of zombie narrative, including the usual free-floating borrowing from plague narrative, the Holocaust, and the militarized inner city of the war on drugs (as we have already frequently seen). This is the story we expect from a zombie comic, after all—a war between the living and the dead. And over the course of the book military figures repeatedly attempt to leap to the genocidal solution, only to be stymied by public opinion, human rights lawyers, or John's inexhaustible decency. And the over-policing, violent suppression, concentration camps, and proposed forced relocation policies are all revealed by the end of *Dead Eyes Open* to be the consequence of misplaced government paranoia, not a genuine threat. In fact, the generals turn out to have been deliberately seeking to *provoke* the sort of violent resistance from the zombies that would justify full-on extermination, without success. This governmental overreach thus becomes the occasion for a civil rights struggle that reveals these proposed policies to be the result of an irrational prejudice against the undead. Zombies, we find out, are people, too: "These are rational beings. These are people . . . facing an unprecedented disability" (chap. 3). Elsewhere in the story, the key "human" characteristic of the zombie is suggested to be not so much its rationality but its continued capacity for love; multiple characters suggest that it is the Returners' love of their families and their desire to remain with them that has caused all this to happen. This is the attitude that prevails at the end of the story: both the zombie-supremacist terrorists and the anti-zombie revanchist shadow government are defeated, clearing the way for integration and inclusion. Liberal tolerance and love thus triumph in the end over hate, dehumanization, and fear, with a zombified Wil Wheaton (of *Star Trek: The Next Generation* fame) announcing his candidacy to be the first Returner governor of California while John embraces his family (including a now-tolerant daughter wearing an "I'm with Wheaton" T-shirt) at the story's close. John could stay in Alaska with many of the other Returners and never rot, perhaps living forever—but he chooses instead to go home to where his loved ones are, no matter how "hard" or "strange" life with his condition will be. "Forever without you," he tells his wife, "isn't a forever I want" (chap. 6). This is a different sort of love than the love that cures the zombie in *Warm Bodies*—because, of course, it is no cure at all. For Shepherd and Boney love is ultimately not what reverses our zombic mortality but rather the force that sustains us and our relationships through it, even as the passing of time inevitably unmakes us all.

The very last page of *Dead Eyes Open* gives some taste of how the world will change to nourish the possibility of a love that can persist in the face of unhappy transformation. This page is a "toe tag" readers can cut out and distribute to support the book, a kind of viral marketing for the project—but it also indicates the kind of zombie ethics of love that here replaces the old zombie ethics of extermination and bitter violence. The layout of the text on the toe tag closely parallels a zombie recruiting poster from earlier in the text that suggested "they believe we are monsters" and called on Returners to "stand up and fight" against their human oppressors (chap. 3). Now that message of violence is reversed: the last page is a call for trust rather than bitter antagonism. This reversal reflects Aquilina and Hughes's (2006, 158) pointed reversal of the usual terms of the zombie metaphor for illness: patients suffering from severe illness, old age, and dementia should be thought of not as "the living dead" but the "dying who live . . . who deserve our care and concern because of their continuing place as persons in the human world." Rather than the shotgun or crowbar that destroys the zombies' broken brain, we find instead in *Dead Eyes Open* a new proposed ethos for zombic medicine: treatment, care, reintegration, love. When zombies can speak, and tell us their stories, and explain their suffering, the fantasy of killing them breaks down, and the circuit of empathy is restored. In the face of a public health crisis like the Returner event—or our own graying society—there must emerge new practices of care and new ways of interacting, but within a logic of inclusion and mutual respect, rather than extermination, elimination, or callous institutionalization. "IF YOU ARE READING THIS TAG YOU ARE A RETURNER," the toe tag reads. "REMAIN CALM. . . . DO NOT ATTEMPT TO HARM YOURSELF OR OTHERS . . . YOU ARE SAFE AND SECURE . . . WELCOME BACK."

NOTES

1. This is more or less my own approach to *The Walking Dead*; see, for instance, my essay "We Are the Walking Dead" (Canavan 2010).
2. Recall that *28 Days Later* was actually filmed primarily *before* September 11, 2001.
3. See, for instance, his foreword to the first trade paperback, *Days Gone Bye* (Kirkman and Moore 2006).
4. This situation was ultimately parodied in a special full-color epilogue to *The Walking Dead* issue 75, in which Rick wakes up (from another coma) to discover he has actually been in precisely *this* sort of alien-invasion story all along.
5. See, for instance, the French series *Les Revenants* (film 2004; television 2012), the BBC series *In the Flesh* (2013), and the film *Life after Beth* (Jeff Baena 2014).
6. Cf. Nixon's discussion of the comic series *Crossed* (2008–10) in this volume.
7. See also the mainline *Blackest Night* series, published by DC at the same time.

8. See especially Iron Man's interrupted attempt at self-reflection in part 2: "I'm starting to forget things. It's starting to become . . ." (Kirkman and Phillips 2005).
9. A similar sense of temporal dislocation is generated by the bizarrely compelling Archie Comics series *Afterlife with Archie* (2014), in which the idyllic permanent-1950s of Riverdale is suddenly shattered by a 2000s-style zombie apocalypse.
10. The slur is a reference to the doctor's ethnic heritage, suggesting the way that in group and out-group dynamics are strongly at work in people's attitudes toward the Revivers. The book as a whole does not endorse ethnocentrism or Islamophobia; the Muslim doctor is actually Dana's primary love interest across the series.
11. The notion is taken from one of the zombie supremacists in the story, whom John kills at the end of chapter 5.

REFERENCES

Aquilina, Carmelo, and Julian C. Hughes. 2006. "The Return of the Living Dead: Agency Lost and Found?" In *Dementia: Mind, Meaning, and the Person*, edited by Julian C. Hughes, Stephen J. Louw, and Steven R. Sabat, 143–61. Oxford, UK: Oxford University Press.

Behuniak, Susan M. 2011. "The Living Dead? The Construction of People with Alzheimer's Disease as Zombies." *Ageing and Society* 31 (1): 70–92.

Beisecker, Dave. 2014. "Afterword: Bye-Gone Days: Reflections on Romero, Kirkman, and What We Become." In *"We're All Infected": Essays on AMC's "The*

Walking Dead" and the Fate of the
Human*, edited by Dawn Keetley, 201–
14. Jefferson, NC: McFarland.

Bunn, Cullen, and Ramon Rosanas. 2014.
Night of the Living Deadpool. Comic
book series. New York: Marvel Comics.

Canavan, Gerry. 2010. "'We Are the Walking
Dead': Race, Time, and Survival in
Zombie Narrative." *Extrapolation* 51 (3):
431–53.

Clarens, Carlos. 1997. *An Illustrated History of
Horror and Science-Fiction Films*. New
York: Da Capo Press.

Ellis, Warren, Max Fiumara, and Ryan Waterhouse. 2007. *Blackgas*. Trade paperback. Rantoul, IL: Avatar Press.

Farnell, Gary. 2014. "'Talking Bodies' in a
Zombie Apocalypse: From the Discursive to the Shitty Sublime." In *"We're All
Infected": Essays on AMC's "The Walking Dead" and the Fate of the Human*,
edited by Dawn Keetley, 173–85. Jefferson, NC: McFarland.

Fitzpatrick, Dan. 2014. "Rising U.S. Life Spans
Spell Likely Pain for Pension Funds."
Wall Street Journal, October 27. http://
www.wsj.com/articles/rising-u-s-life
spans-spell-likely-pain-for-pension
-funds-1414430683.

Herskovits, Elizabeth. 1995. "Struggling over
Subjectivity: Debates about the 'Self'
and Alzheimer's Disease." *Medical
Anthropology Quarterly* 9 (2): 146–64.

Johns, Geoff, and Ivan Reis. 2009–10. *Blackest
Night: The Flash*. Comic book series.
New York: DC Comics.

Johnston, Rich. 2012. "*The Walking Dead*
Alien Invasion That Never Was: Robert Kirkman at Image Comics Expo."
Bleeding Cool, February 17. http://
www.bleedingcool.com/2012/02/27/
the-walking-dead-alien-invasion-that

-never-was-robert-kirkman-at-image
-comics-expo/.

Kirkman, Robert, and Tony Moore. 2006. *Days
Gone Bye*. Trade paperback. Berkeley,
CA: Image Comics.

Kirkman, Robert, Tony Moore, and Charlie
Adlard. 2003–. *The Walking Dead*.
Comic book series. Berkeley, CA:
Image Comics.

Kirkman, Robert, and Sean Phillips. 2005.
Marvel Zombies. Trade paperback. New
York: Marvel Comics.

Lauro, Sarah Juliet, and Karen Embry. 2008.
"A Zombie Manifesto: The Nonhuman
Condition in the Era of Advanced Cap-
italism." *boundary 2* 35 (1): 85–108.

"Old Europe." 2004. *The Economist*, September
30. http://www.economist.com/
node/3243014.

Panda, Ankit. 2014. "Japan's Demographic Crisis: Any Way Out?" *The Diplomat*,
March 26. http://thediplomat.
com/2014/03/japans-demographic-
crisis-any-way-out.

Reyes, Xavier Aldana. 2014. "Nothing but the
Meat: Posthuman Bodies and the
Dying Undead." In *"We're All Infected":
Essays on AMC's "The Walking Dead"
and the Fate of the Human*, edited by
Dawn Keetley, 142–55. Jefferson, NC:
McFarland.

Seeley, Tim, and Mike Norton. 2012–. *Revival*.
Comic book series. Berkeley, CA:
Image Comics.

Shepherd, Matthew, and Roy Boney, Jr. 2005.
Dead Eyes Open. Trade paperback. San
Jose: SLG.

Williams, Timothy. 2014. "Graying of America
Is Speeding, Report Says." *New York
Times*, May 6. http://www.nytimes.
com/2014/05/07/us/graying-of-america
-is-speeding-report-says.html.

2.

VIRAL VIRULENCE, POSTMODERN ZOMBIES, AND THE AMERICAN HEALTHCARE ENTERPRISE IN THE ANTIBIOTIC AGE

Kari Nixon

The formula: Find the microbe and kill it. And even
that [scientists] did not know how to do.
—George Bernard Shaw,
The Doctor's Dilemma, 1906

In a world where bacterial infections have been temporarily sapped of their power, viruses now threaten postmodern man in a way that bacteria no longer can. The virus sits on the liminal line of existence, silently yet insistently challenging our most basic assumptions about the categories that make up life and death, animate and inanimate, thereby worrying away at the boundaries of individual and national identity. This essay explores the medical and scientific discourse packaged into current representations of zombies (another image of liminal life) by overlaying this cultural phenomenon with the concerns of vitality raised by viruses, especially in light of recent shifts in the tropes and conventions deployed in media that portray zombie pandemics. Most prominently and of importance in this essay, the viral infection has become associated with zombiism. I argue that if the trope of the virus toys with the tensile strength of the binaries that define life and death, the human and inhuman, then recent graphic narratives about zombies put pressure on the binarisms that facilitate American private healthcare practices. These binarisms, as I discuss them here, are often constructed to define categories such as sick versus well, what groups are worthy of medical care, and are necessary to sustain an economically unsustainable approach to healthcare. As Atul Gawande (2009) has famously noted in "The Cost Conundrum," "Universal [health] coverage won't be feasible unless we can control costs," but "Americans like to believe that, with most things, more is better," even though evidence mostly suggests the contrary in regard to expensive medical testing. As it is, expensive care mandates the selection of specific groups that can afford this care, and this selection criteria often rests on financial means or, relatedly, employment in privileged jobs that provide generous insurance benefits. Thus this essay explores the ways that the graphic media of zombie comics pair image and text in unique ways that work to critique the systemic infrastructures that inscribe American (and, by symbolic implication, international) bodies with constructed difference while vividly depicting their sameness. The cognitive dissonance between these two dynamics, particularly when represented in still-frame graphic renderings and graphically displayed textual features, works to destabilize readers' sense that what makes an epidemic is clear-cut, that what marks the ill is obvious, and it exposes the American healthcare system as one that relies on segregation and separatism for its survival.

Recent graphic renderings of zombie apocalypses have brought the concerns of this viral vector to bear on its human protagonists. Two in particular blur the lines between the ostensibly stable categories of human/not-human, infected/not-infected, and zombie/not-zombie. Simultaneously and perhaps more insistently, the universal viral infection depicted in *The Walking Dead* (Kirkman, Moore, and Adlard 2003–) as well as the selective infection in *Crossed* (Ennis 2008–10) both destabilize the perception that only biological factors (such as r-noughts and signs/symptoms of infection) define epidemics and our responses to them.[1] I argue that in *The Walking Dead* the universal infection combined with graphic juxtapositions of similarly maimed human and "nonhuman" bodies leave no room for physiological differences between the groups defined as sick and well, while medical treatment of these two groups is vastly different—as different, say, as first-world Americans and their impoverished counterparts here and abroad. In my analysis of *Crossed* I move on to explore how cognitive alterities operate under a similar infrastructure, as both the American Psychiatric Association, proprietor of the *Diagnostic and Statistical Manual of Mental Disorders* (*DSM*), and American health insurance companies rely on diagnostic bifurcations of cognitive states for their fiscal survival. *Crossed* does not implicate universal infection but rather a more typical distinction between the infected and the noninfected as it paradoxically and simultaneously concocts an "illness" that is revealed to be no different from "normative" human nature.

As readers our sense of universal infection (or in the case of *Crossed*, universal non-normality) has become pressing as we approach problematic biomedical challenges. On the one hand, due to the increased and now ubiquitous use of antibiotics since their inception, bacteria have evolved to resist even our most potent antibiotics, in many cases leaving us defenseless. On the other, though biomedicine has developed some treatments against viruses, such as antiretrovirals, the nature of viral replication and evolution within hosts and between species poses continued obstacles to researchers and practitioners.

While Bernard Shaw's adage "Find the microbe and kill it" has long since been realized in the realm of bacterial infections, the same sort of seek-and-destroy imperative that biomedicine so fervently deploys has been contested as we now confront the question of how to kill that which is not living—how to confront, that is, that which challenges our most basic assumptions of national and individual subjectivity and existence alongside the systems we have constructed to sustain them.

Zombies in *Crossed* are virally infected with a contagion that releases the Freudian id from the shackles of the superego, as it were—in the worst ways imaginable. Rather than mindless, shambling hordes, typical of zombie fiction and featured in *The Walking Dead*, zombies in *Crossed* are often calculating and manipulative in their violence and purposefully inflict as much trauma and pain on their victims as possible. Juxtaposition of these two series allows for consideration of the liminality of existence rendered visible by viral pathogens. What is it exactly that the virus threatens: physical sentience, moral and empathetic potential, or something broader? Can we "*be* without borders," as Kristeva asked long ago? That is, can there be meaning in a medicalized world where our physical and psychic vulnerability is all too obvious? In seeking to answer these questions, I move now to explore how authors and illustrators exploit the liminal space of virality to probe the depths of the binaristic constructs that sustain our modern medical and psychiatric enterprises, enterprises that deeply define our sense of the normative and worthy body and mind.

Recent zombie narratives such as the films *28 Days Later* (Danny Boyle 2003) and *World War Z* (Marc Forster 2013) have relied on viral infection as the vector of both contagion and plot.[2] In fact, I would argue that virally transmitted zombie plagues are so ubiquitous to the genre that in many of the more current renditions seen since the emergence of the "zombie craze" (circa 2009) the viral nature of this pathogen has become such a common trope as to often go unstated and simply assumed within narrative bounds. In fact, both of the comics I discuss here zip past epidemiologically chronicling the infection to focus on its aftermath and reshaping of the meanings and definitions of the "well" human. Both *Crossed* and *The Walking Dead* skip questions of transmission that have been rather set in stone by generic conventions—such as the cause of zombiism being a pathogen that follows recognizable epidemiological parameters like air- or saliva-borne transmission—in order, I would argue, to focus the heft of their story lines on more prescient biopolitical questions.[3] It is this very tropological reliance on a sort of human-vectored rabies (*28 Days Later* is most obvious in this regard, terming its imaginary viral agent the "rage virus," hearkening to the furious stage of rabies viral infections) that exposes zombie films' preoccupation with the boundaries of the human. Rabies, after all, has been since the nineteenth century largely a disease of *non*human animals, who were and still are simply euthanized rather than treated, and, as previously noted, viruses call into question the limits of meaningful organic life altogether. Considering that rabies—or any infection via bite wound—is actually a rather inefficient way of spreading a global epidemic (as opposed to, say, respiratory infections), the phenomenological implications of this viral bite wound infection, with its historical links to *non*human actors, bear consideration in terms of what medical discourses are inscribed, repurposed, or reimagined in a genre that relies so heavily on this imaginative and rather unrealistic mode of contamination.

As the maimed bodies of *The Walking Dead* survivors dwindle to their most essential parts—eyes, hands, and feet lost along the way—their discernible differences from decaying and maimed zombie bodies dwindle as well, leaving only a mass of human and "once-human" bodies, all equally marked by the collective violence of their situation. The increasingly identical bodies of the humans and the zombies force readers to consider biopolitical questions of who exactly we deem worth treating in times of epidemic, which then leads to uncomfortable questions about the *non*-epidemiological factors that affect epidemic spread—factors such as access to care, the function of media publicity in care, and other social biases affecting not only who is eligible for care but also whom we call "infected." This last point is especially tangible in *The Walking Dead* since the universal infection of all human and "once-human" bodies is a major turning point of the narrative. Thus the humble virus is the universal leveler that yokes human bodies together in a universal state of infection, disallowing points of pure biology to act as a means of categorical binarism. More poignantly, nearly to the point of black comedy, the comic's miraculously ever-present medics, all scrambling to sew worthy bodies back together, set the questions of access to and worthiness of care in even higher contrast. As the creator Robert Kirkman notes in his preface to the series, "how these characters get" where they are "is more important" than the action of them "getting there"; in a real biopolitical sense, then, the road that led to our current profit-based healthcare system is a question well worth asking according to this series.

The first issue of *The Walking Dead* famously opens with Rick in a hospital bed recovering from a gunshot wound. Thus the series begins with an illustration of a prostrate, injured human body, already not so very different from the shambling hordes of "nonhuman" bodies on which the genre predicates itself. Importantly, the very first zombie Rick sees falls helplessly out of an elevator when Rick opens the door, staring motionlessly up at him, mouth agape. The confrontation of injured body with injured body, graphically rendered and connected, sets the tone for a series less about human conquering of nonhuman, but rather about the cognitive leaps necessary for the individual to sustain his false categorical separation of himself from the zombies who are rather like him. As Žižek (2008) has noted, physical violence often serves merely to mask the systemic violence that has caused its eruption, and in these very first panels of *The Walking Dead*, readers are confronted with two equally infected bodies, both injured and staggering about. Like the dividing practices of privatized healthcare, which decide which lives are worth saving and which can be left to die, the zombie genre insists on fundamental differences between the two—between the valued human and the abject zombie—for its perpetuation. Showing Rick's face inches away from the first zombie he witnesses, the panel emphasizes their similarities rather than their differences: both of their mouths stand awkwardly agape, their disheveled, unshorn faces mirror each other, and both lie prone on the floor, the space between them connected by Rick's realization of their similar plight as he frantically calls for help for what he initially interprets as another victim of injury or illness just like himself.

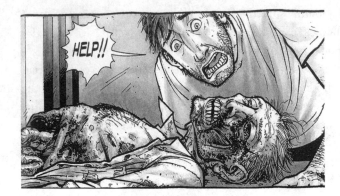

2.1 Rick's elevator encounter from *The Walking Dead*. Illustrated by Tony Moore.

Shortly thereafter, a second zombie tackles him but succeeds only in falling and breaking his own feeble neck. In fact, Rick and the Stairway Zombie actually fall together, once more underscoring their similarly fragile human corporeal structures rather than their fundamental differences via visual juxtaposition. As they land on the floor, the cell highlights in freeze-frame their entangled bodies, both similarly flailing, and both similarly injured by their fall. Rick happens to emerge victorious from this scuffle not because of his "human" status, but simply based on the coincidence of the position in which he falls. The third individual zombie Rick encounters after exiting the hospital (the famed "Bicycle Girl") has decayed to the point of being a mere skeleton. She stares up at Rick and groans helplessly. Her languid body, situated next to a wrecked bike, is arranged as any human body might be after a mere fall from a vehicle. As she stares at Rick the visual tone is undoubtedly one of sympathy.

In this famous scene, readers are first witness to what I argue is one of the comic's major devices emphasizing similarities between zombie and human bodies. Small panels lined neatly in a row show first Rick's face then the girl's in repeated sequence. In this particular instance Rick's initial awareness of the humanity of the zombies—so similar to his own injured body—is highlighted. However, on a broader level, depictions like this function to physically link the sets of bodies in a way that purely textual or filmic media could not. Although shot / reverse shot might be a comparable method in film, the black lines that separate these panels, so typical of *The Walking Dead*, provide a more literal juxtaposition of images, connecting and yet dividing them simultaneously, illustrating vividly the cognitive dissonance between imagined difference and actual similarity that the series is invested in critiquing.

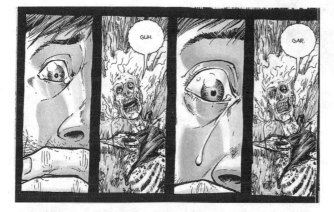

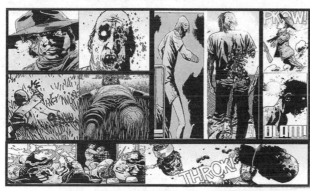

As the series continues the alternating panel layout is used more frequently, often to pair the humans' reliance on denying this unity by physically separating themselves from the zombies with an array of fortresses. Yet, throughout the series, the maimed bodies of humans and zombies accrue enormously, and this host of bodies—all linked in infection despite the imaginative borders they erect around themselves—is depicted via counterpart juxtaposition. It is in fact difficult to find a human injury not mimicked by a zombie in the series.

Moreover, whereas still-frame panels repeating nearly identical images carry out the theme of emphasizing the piteousness of the injured human body, it is sound effects—graphically rendered—that serve to tabulate the ever-accruing number of bodies deemed not worthy of treatment, also known as zombies. Both devices are served by the graphic novel medium as sound effects in film tend to fade into the background, whereas the various "thawks" and "pows" in *The Walking Dead* ring in the visual memory of the reader, rendering the unworthiness of the bodies therein more palpable.

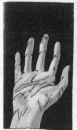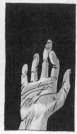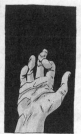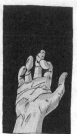

2.4 Repeated, consecutive images of an injured human hand from *The Walking Dead*. Illustrated by Charlie Adlard.

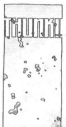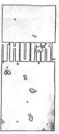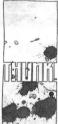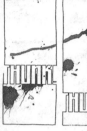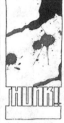

2.5 Repeated, consecutive, graphically rendered sound effects, which often represent killed zombie bodies, from *The Walking Dead*. Illustrated by Charlie Adlard.

These sound effects and visual repeats force the reader's awareness of the sheer number of moments focused on injured human bodies and killed zombie ones in a way that a lingering shot or background sound effect could not. Both bodies remain similarly infected and similarly injured—but their treatment is vastly different, even in this graphic medium.

Thus, as the series insistently indicates, there is nothing physically different between the two groups. However, the "human" group *must* themselves insist on this difference if they are to survive. No one could reasonably argue that to save or treat all the zombies is a sustainable practice—a fact illustrated by Rick and Hershel's famous argument over the zombies Hershel has kept in the barn. In volume 2, issue 11 (Kirkman, Moore, and Adlard 2003–), after Carl's shooting, the group meets Hershel, a retired veterinarian who heals Carl and later reveals to Rick that he is one of the only people who has thought to treat the infected people as infected *people*.[4] He explains to Rick that he is keeping the zombies he finds in his barn "until we can figure out a way to help them," and then seems surprised that one would do anything else. "What have you been doing with them?" he asks Rick, who responds that they have of course "been killing them." A heated argument follows, during which Herschel points out that Rick has taken the allocation of medical treatment on himself. The zombies, he points out, "don't come with an instruction manual," highlighting the unknown nature of the causal pathogen that infects them. He continues: "We don't know a goddamn thing about them. We don't know what they're thinking—what they're feeling," rendering bare the seemingly naturalized assumptions that perpetuate zombie media as unthinking hedonistic fulfillment of violent desires rather than focusing on the always-present pathogenic illness that lies behind this corporeal change. Although Hershel makes several very worthy biopolitical arguments regarding the import of attempting to treat the zombies as one would any other infected patient, he quickly abandons this moral ship when the zombies break out and nearly kill him.

Here is the crux of the issue represented in *The Walking Dead*'s style: the system of American medical practices *cannot* sustainably treat everyone, and therefore relies on superficial differences (in our real-world economic striations, in the series-world false corporeal binaries) to sift out a small subsection of the population deemed worthy of treating with limited and irresponsibly allocated resources. Its aforementioned reliance on comparative links between zombie and human pushes back against this capitalistic enterprise as the series insists on the actual likeness between the two groups, while simultaneously holding in tension that the system as it stands actually *cannot* viably support both. The system itself must be razed to the ground, the series seems to suggest, even as it coyly hints that the American ethos of capitalistic exclusion is such a firmly established zeitgeist that even an apocalypse serves only to reconstruct such strictures in a rudimentary fashion. The odd and rather unrealistic presence of doctors throughout the series, assiduously working to stitch together the bodies they see as worthy of treatment, make this abundantly clear. While Hershel's plan of preserving zombie bodies for eventual care is instantly revealed as ineffective, medical treatment is available in the privileged survivor communities that are somehow always decently equipped with medical supplies, clean linens, and comfortable beds. All of these provisions bleakly expose the dubious inequalities between the two groups of afflicted human bodies and give a ring of satire to the series through its sheer unlikelihood. Even when Rick is in the clutches of the villainous Governor character, he is given access to rather sophisticated medical care. In speaking of "basic" medical supplies such as gauze, bandages, and clean linens, the first-world mind is reminded mostly of advertisements for charitable organizations that provide such equipment to third-world countries. The privileged access to such items in the world of the comic once again hearkens to systemic inequalities and turn Rick Grimes's famous statement, "WE are the walking dead," back toward readers themselves, most likely the very privileged individuals of our world's version of these inequities.

Like *The Walking Dead*, *Crossed* begins in medias res, and questions of infectious vectors are allowed to rest on the zombie genre's conventions. Once again, just as the generically conventional virus hovers in the imaginative background of the zombie framework, complicating the border between life and death, so do the zombie figures in *Crossed* serve to disrupt the boundaries of human subjectivity and consider the *non*-epidemiological factors that we use to separate the well from the sick. The major generic diversion of *Crossed* is that it creates perhaps the first-ever representation of thinking, calculating zombies, thus moving the crosshairs of biopolitical consideration from purely corporeal manifestations of illness to cognitive indicators. In fact, the so-called zombies in *Crossed* arguably think more than their human victims do. Issue 0, "Prologue" (Ennis 2008–10), begins with a reference to contemporary viral video culture. The first speech frame of the series simply asks, "Remember YouTube?" before going on to note that the first accounts of the zombie attacks in this world were through videos gone viral, all met with a ubiquitous world response of "Fake!" (issue 0). The narrator explains that most people gave the viral videos of viral infection "no thought" because humanity had become "unshockable" through its own capacity for malicious and violent acts. Yet, much like the imagined binaries between sets of bodies in *The Walking Dead*, it is the very malicious violence of the zombies in *Crossed* that supposedly demarcates them from their human counterparts. The narrator continues: "Nothing was real, because nothing affected us, not our war, not the planet coughing blood and quitting. We absorbed or we ignored." Consistent with most zombie narratives, the viral infection is an assumed convention that lingers in the series, and *Crossed* thus begins with reference to the more prominent form of virality that defines our digital age. Moreover, the narrator argues, it is this technological virality that has allowed for the viral spread of our own vicious impulses and has duly rendered *us* the unthinking, shambling zombies, incapable of feeling affect when faced with zombies that are more thinking and feeling (albeit in a sadistic direction) than we are. As the first zombie enters the frame of the narrator, dropping a half-torn human spine onto the counter of the diner where he sits, the nonreactive faces of the diner patrons set the backdrop for the narrator's commentary: in this disillusioned postmodern culture, no one had any idea that "something *real* was coming." If nothing from YouTube documentation had been deemed "real," the series suggests, the breakdown of mind-numbing digital virality and the introduction of pathogenic virality ushers in an era of palpable reality, where humans are forced to confront a nightmarish pandemic of the rapists and murderers

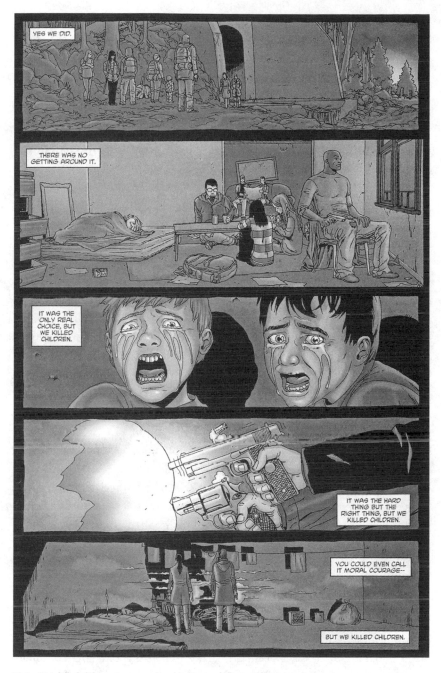

2.6 "We killed children," contemplated in *Crossed*. Illustrated by Jacen Burrows.

to and by whom it has become desensitized. "The truth we wanted," in a fragmented postmodernity, the narrator remarks, "was exactly what we didn't want to face" (issue 4). Namely, if loss of cognition supposedly defines the *non*human zombie, then the ostensibly humanized, thinking zombies in *Crossed* bring devastating implications to bear on the supposed sanctity of humanity.

If *The Walking Dead* provocatively asks us to evaluate who the walking dead really are, not just in the series but in our own setting, wherein third-world countries are as deprived of basic medical equipment as are the zombies in the series, *Crossed* asks readers to consider our defining criteria of cognitive alterity in an intimately interconnected world. Where is alterity to be situated, exactly, in a world with increasingly invisible boundaries? Moreover, the series again provokes questions regarding access to care in a cosmos where zombies and humans are often shown to be equally as malicious.

The lengths to which the characters will go in brutalizing other humans simply to avoid becoming the somehow fundamentally more evil Crossed hearkens hauntingly to present-day vaccination debates, in which the horror of autism—a cognitive state somehow beyond the pale, the terrors of which are yet somehow a social given—is so patently untenable that physical disease and epidemic is preferable. As with *The Walking Dead*, repeated language and images in *Crossed*'s panels is often used to make this point. The most apt example of this occurs when the "protagonist" group kills a class of children they believe will slow them down in escaping the violent Crossed. As the narrator contemplates his actions in hindsight, his inner monologue is written repeatedly in each panel: "We killed children." Like the sound effects in *The Walking Dead*, these sentences accrue numerically and, when paired with the repeated images of the terrified faces of the murdered children, serve to veritably tally the acts of the so-called cognitively normal humans against those of the altered mental state of the Crossed.

Crossed similarly castigates a social system that has both created unchecked mental violence in its populace as well as fostered a sense of elitism through categorization of mental states via manuals such as the *DSM*, now in its fifth edition. The series exposes human "morality" as but a frail palimpsest justifying a biopolitical framework that upholds profit and separatism to maintain itself. Indeed, the narrator notes that one might consider the murder of the children a form of "moral courage," thereby highlighting, as *The Walking Dead* does via visual representations of supposed corporeal boundaries, the imagined mental differences applied to the same acts that separate the mentally "well" from the mentally "ill."

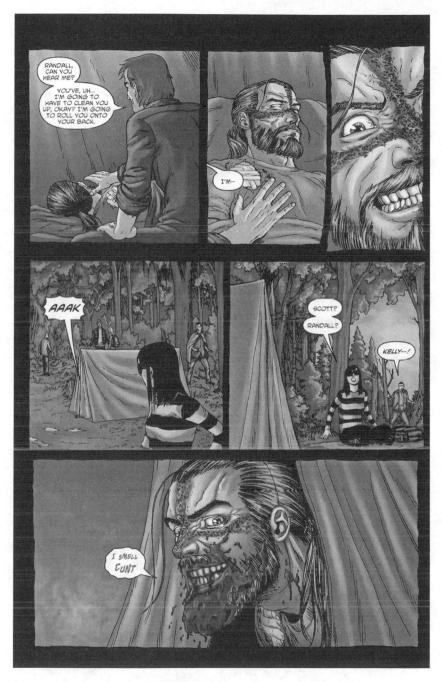

2.7 The hashed face of the Crossed. Illustrated by Jacen Burrows.

Although the zombies in the series are described as "crossed" because of odd hash marks that appear on the faces of the infected, the title of the series broaches the precise subject of what it means to "cross" the line of humanity and the inhumane, and whether this "inhumanity" necessarily indicates a descent into the realm of the animalistic—or something worse. Like *The Walking Dead*, the implication of *Crossed* acts to destabilize the human/animal boundary by implying that hierarchical terms such as "animalistic" are meaningless in a world defined by a humanity far more depraved than that allowed for by previous centuries of human philosophy. However, in both graphic narratives the intrinsic viral connection between human and zombie—here rendered in high contrast in the comic's first panels as a networked viral connectivity responsible for the disillusionment of the human race—blurs the line between the two supposedly disparate species. Moreover, the vivid facial cross-marks reiterate the false cognitive binaries implicit in the American psychiatric system by echoing visually the language of the *DSM* itself, which operates via a checklist-style mode of diagnosis (e.g., "indicated by at least 5 of the 9 following symptoms"). One can imagine psychiatric diagnosticians checking off the subsequent boxes next to the bulleted list of symptoms—or, as the case may be, marking them with cross-like hash marks as they categorize the unique subjectivity of their patients which, whether they like it or not, is mandated for insurance reimbursement. Ultimately, the narrator's main insight at the volume's conclusion is bleak: "There was no great secret to the Crossed. I'd never seen one do anything a human being couldn't think of doing. . . . They were all the awful aspects of humanity magnified a hundred-thousandfold but they were nothing more" (issue 9). By yoking the entire species to a universe of contamination that destabilizes all the comforting binaries and hierarchies that ossify the human as something discrete and superior, both series suggest that we, at least, have had our chance and have done a poor job with it. Finding the causal microbe of human downfall, it would seem, is a fruitless effort, for if we were to pinpoint it, we would likely be looking in the mirror.

NOTES

1. R-nought refers to how contagious a disease is by defining how many new cases of infection spawn from one case.
2. Although Dawn Keetley (2014, 3) notes that the zombie apocalypse in *Night of the Living Dead* (George Romero 1968) is

"explained vaguely as the result of radiation from a Venus probe," she and others nevertheless assert that Romero introduced the "infected zombie" trope by depicting zombies who transform others through bite wounds. Steven Pokornowski (2014, 42) similarly notes "the marriage of flesh-eating zombies with medicalized causes is often seen as having its inception with *Night of the Living Dead.*"

3. Dave Beisecker (2014, 202) notes, "*The Walking Dead* skips over the real beginning. Perhaps that is because it has become all too familiar to us. We live in an age in which we don't need to be told . . . how to handle the undead."

4. Pokornowski (2014) and Reyes (2014) also discuss Hershel's ethics in this scene.

REFERENCES

Beisecker, Dave. 2014. "Afterword: Bye-Gone Days: Reflections on Romero, Kirkman, and What We Become." In *"We're All Infected": Essays on AMC's "The Walking Dead" and the Fate of the Human,* edited by Dawn Keetley, 201–14. Jefferson, NC: McFarland.

Ennis, Garth. 2008–10. *Crossed.* Comic book series. Rantoul, IL: Avatar Press.

Gawande, Atul. 2009. "The Cost Conundrum." *New Yorker,* June 1. http://www.new yorker.com/magazine/2009/06/01/ the-cost-conundrum.

Keetley, Dawn. 2014. "Introduction." In *"We're All Infected": Essays on AMC's "The Walking Dead" and the Fate of the Human,* edited by Dawn Keetley, 3–27. Jefferson, NC: McFarland.

Kirkman, Robert, Tony Moore, and Charlie Adlard. 2003–. *The Walking Dead.* Comic book series. Berkeley, CA: Image Comics.

Pokornowski, Steven. 2014. "Burying the Living with the Dead: Security, Survival, and the Sanction of Violence." In *"We're All Infected": Essays on AMC's "The Walking Dead" and the Fate of the Human,* edited by Dawn Keetley, 41–55. Jefferson, NC: McFarland.

Reyes, Xavier Aldana. 2014. "Nothing but the Meat: Posthuman Bodies and the Dying Undead." In *"We're All Infected": Essays on AMC's "The Walking Dead" and the Fate of the Human,* edited by Dawn Keetley, 142–55. Jefferson, NC: McFarland.

Žižek, Slavoj. 2008. *Violence: Six Sideways Reflections.* New York: Picador.

3.

"THE CURE HAS KILLED US ALL"

Dramatizing Medical Ethics Through Zombie and Period Fiction Tropes in *The New Deadwardians*

Tully Barnett and Ben Kooyman

The figure of the zombie carries death and decay into a world obsessed with medical healing and health. Zombies, as they exist in contemporary popular culture, are an illness taken to its extreme, one that is highly infectious and cannot be healed. Moreover, tales of reanimated bodies, from Mary Shelley's *Frankenstein* (1818) through to *The Walking Dead* (comic 2003–; television 2010–) have long articulated topical concerns around medical science, scientific hubris, the abuse of knowledge and power, and the boundaries between the living and the dead. Fiction set in earlier periods, the Edwardian period in this case, likewise enables discourse on our contemporary concerns through processes of comparison, contrast, analogy, metaphor, and defamiliarization. As Jerome de Groot (2009, 3) notes, "History is other and the present familiar," and this Otherness provides a means of examining the familiar with fresh insights and perspectives. Bringing the two modes of zombie and historical narrative together, then, creates a space to consider the medicalization of the human and the potential for misuse underpinning the creation and dissemination of medical assets and resources.

This chapter examines the comic series *The New Deadwardians* (2012; trade paperback, 2013), written by Dan Abnett and illustrated by I. N. J. Culbard, and discusses the relationship between illness, medicalization, class, and location in this work. The series is set in the aftermath of a zombie outbreak, where the authorities and upper and middle classes utilize a medical cure that transforms them into vampiric beings in order to conquer the zombie population. While infection and survival are key preoccupations of most zombie narratives, dramatizing concerns about infection and fear of pandemics, this narrative centers on the treatment of the condition and, more important, its long-term impact on a reconstituted society. Its focus thus is what Priscilla Wald (2008, 17) calls "the institutional legacy of communicable disease, the policies and practices set in place to prevent or manage devastating outbreaks." This focus is consistent with historical chronicles of illness and epidemic which, as Wald notes, focused on how it "ravaged the social order as much as it did individual bodies" (11). Those familiar with zombie narratives will recognize these motifs, and *The New Deadwardians* joins a growing body of zombie works concerned not only with survival but with scenarios of cohabitation alongside and reconstruction of society around the zombie threat, including films such as *Land of the Dead* (George Romero 2005), *Fido* (Andrew Currie 2006), *Warm Bodies* (Jonathan Levine 2013), and *Life after Beth* (Jeff Baena 2014). *The New Deadwardians* adopts a pessimistic attitude toward rehabilitation and reconciliation. While the medical cure prolongs the lives of the public and is created for the "good" of society, it does not actually "cure" zombiism and indeed generates social unrest due to the unjust distribution of therapeutic intervention. Further, this treatment erodes the humanity of those who take it—hence, as one character reflects, "The Cure has killed us all" (issue 6, p. 17).

The use of zombie and vampire archetypes enables commentary on the negative consequences of misusing medical knowledge and resources, as does the setting in an alternate version of Edwardian England. The story frequently evokes and gently subverts touchstones of this era, as well as its precursor, the Victorian age. Edwardian class structure is associated with different types of creatures—zombies with the poor and lower working class, vampires with the aristocracy and upwardly mobile middle class, accentuating the inequity of ownership and control of medical assets. Edwardian London was the superpower of one hundred years past, and hence it generates parallels with and enables critique of today's United States and its inequitable distribution of medical knowledge and resources. In considering medicalization in zombie narratives, we follow Peter Conrad (2008, 4), who sees medicalization as "a process by which nonmedical problems become defined and treated as medical problems." The series comments on the alignment of lower classes with death and disease and the upper classes with health and cleanliness. Furthermore, given the narrative's reinforcement of the Edwardian status quo through the use of the Cure, it is consistent with a medical tradition in which "the bodies of white, European, middle-class, heterosexual men have been constructed as the standard for measuring and evaluating other bodies" (Alan Petersen, cited in Conrad 2008, 24).

The intentions of this chapter are threefold. First, it examines the depiction in *The New Deadwardians* of the abuse of medical knowledge and how this misuse fuels social discontent. Second, it elucidates the text's thesis that this misuse of medical assets is detrimental to and ultimately destroys both those who wield them (the vampiric upper and upper middle classes) and those who do not (the lower middle and working classes who lack access to the Cure, and the infected zombie lower class). Health or lack thereof aligns sharply with class in a manner that mirrors recent concerns around access to health benefits and resources. Finally, the chapter identifies correspondences between these themes and our contemporary condition, highlighting the use of period setting and zombie and horror tropes in *The New Deadwardians* as an effective means for dramatizing ethical concerns around access to medical assets. The text is ultimately somewhat superficial in its treatment of these issues, and asks more questions than it answers; nonetheless, its treatment of these issues is worth exploring.

The Restless Curse: Edwardian Epidemic

The New Deadwardians presents an alternate history of Edwardian England, imagining this era as it exists after a zombie outbreak. Set in 1910, the series follows Inspector Suttle's investigation of the murder of an aristocrat in an age supposedly post-death. We learn that fifty years previously, in the 1860s, zombielike creatures known as "the Restless" arose and ravaged England and the globe. The ruling class—law enforcers and officers in the Memorial War army—and those in positions of wealth or authority were provided with a medicinal intervention known as "the Cure" and became creatures known as "the Young," beings who resemble vampires and are invisible to the Restless (because they are similarly lifeless). The split between the Young and the Restless falls across class lines.[1] The Young are predominantly England's ruling class, while the Restless inhabit the fringes of society, abject and *Other*; those neither Young nor Restless—normal humans who are born, age, die, and display the normal appetites of human life—are known as "the Bright" and occupy the lower middle and working underclass and are relegated to a special area of London called Zone B. These class divisions inform who has access to and control of medicine and how that benefit is disseminated. The Bright, because they lack access to the Cure, are disempowered and constantly under threat of death or infection by zombie attack. Moreover, the close connection between class structure and the geographical spaces of London reinforces the cultural stereotype of the East End as diseased. Paul Newland (2008, 39–40) points out that while originally the eastern part of the city was a respite from the urbanity of central London, at least as far back as Daniel Defoe's *A Journal of the Plague Year* there has been a tendency to see the area that would become known as the East End as a dirty and diseased space. For Newland, "the East End of London has often been discussed within the discourse of degeneration and regeneration—discourses which, of course, offer ways of seeing both the human body and the body of the city" (15). The era in which the zombie plague was generated—the 1860s—and that in which the story takes place—the 1910s—are both times of rapid advancement of medical knowledge, some of which reinforced this stereotype.

Zombiism is depicted in *The New Deadwardians* as an infectious disease spread by contact. It is a disease that terminates the life (and humanity) of the infected and of any others the infected kills. The cause of the original outbreak is unknown for much of the story, and various accounts and explanations of its emergence are provided. For example, Suttle recalls early in the story, "We don't know where the Restless Curse came from. A plague, of a form unknown to science. Perhaps an ancient pathogenic bacillus released from the depths of the Earth. It was 1861, the year Poor Prince Albert died. There was a terrible earthquake in Sumatra that year. Or was it just a gypsy curse? A witch's hex? No less likely than a bacillus" (issue 2, p. 6).

The 1860s were a time of growth in knowledge about pathogens, including Rudolph Virchow's work on cellular pathology, which initially conflicted with but eventually became compatible with Louis Pasteur's germ theory. Virchow's view of diseased tissue being caused by a breakdown of order at a cellular level resonates with discourses of social control, as does Pasteur's view about disease being caused due to invasion by foreign organisms. The infection of a populace by an outbreak of zombification reflects such microbiological infection, and the series also connects infection to colonialism, underscoring the link between medical and social concerns. Elsewhere, Suttle's assistant Bowes suggests the disease was brought back from colonial conflicts overseas: "My old mum, she said it was magic. Some heathen hocus-pocus brought back from India or the Afghan wars. She always reckoned we had no business being out there. She said we had a nice country here, why did we need to go blithering around in Johnny Foreignland building an empire" (issue 4, p. 20).

Such speculative accounts paint a portrait of a superpower crippled by infection and disease. The imagery of zombies as primary antagonists and the embodiment of disease is fitting, as the idea of apocalypse structures both social breakdown and infectious outbreak. As Wald (2008, 1) notes of the SARS scare of the 2000s, "The question simmering beneath even the most sedate of accounts was whether this disease . . . might be 'the coming plague' . . . the species-threatening event forecast by scientists and journalists and dramatized in fiction and film in the closing decades of the twentieth century."

Much research has been done on this intersection between colonialism and disease. Warwick Anderson (1995) and Alison Bashford (2000) study the imperialistic perspectives prevalent in the study of tropical medicine in the late nineteenth and early twentieth centuries where "bacteriology's colonial enthusiasts eagerly sought out, isolated, and disinfected native reservoirs and transmitters of pathology" (Anderson 1995, 644). For Anderson in his analysis of the role of health imagery in the relationship between the United States and the Philippines, "American bodily control legitimated and symbolized social and political control" (643) and "the new tropical medicine thus provides an instance of a material power that operates on distinctly racial bodies to produce the sort of body that colonial society required" (645). Texts written by colonists in Africa in the nineteenth century use the term "hordes," evoking the peoples of Africa in a way similar to descriptions of zombie hordes (for example, see Philip 1828). Images of colonial misdeeds pervade Culbard's art: as Suttle recalls this history early in the story he stares at an antiquated military recruitment poster on his superior officer's wall (issue 2, p. 6), while his later conversation with Bowes is peppered with flashbacks to his military days battling the zombies, wearing the same iconic red uniform sported by Michael Caine, Stanley Baker, and others in the Cy Endfield film *Zulu* (1964). The comic book's images put the zombies in the position of the Zulus in both Endfield's film and historical reality, reinforcing the association between zombies and Zulus as uncivilized *Others* to be annihilated by the Empire, just as diseases are to be eradicated.

By aligning the zombies with the Zulu people at the time of the Anglo-Zulu War (1879), the authors draw explicit connections between exploitative treatment of the peoples of Africa under colonial rule and the disenfranchised Londoners of the East End, who either become zombies or are vulnerable to zombie attack. *The New Deadwardians* thus draws parallels between zombie horror and historical fears of the Other.[2] The zombie is an ideal vehicle for this symbolism, having embodied the potential horrors of both exotic, distant locales—best exemplified in *White Zombie* (Victor Halperin 1932)—and the threat posed by the lower classes at home—best exemplified in George Romero's zombie films, where the creatures are typically "blue-collar monsters" (Inguanzo 2014, 16). There are also, however, connotations of justice to be found in the infection of the colonizers: given that their pathogens destroyed many indigenous communities, images of the colonized returning from the grave and turning on the Empire that decimated them carry a hint of poetic justice, as well as echoing Freud's notion of the return of the repressed.[3]

However, Suttle's investigation ultimately reveals that the source of the Restless Curse was a spell cast by the dark magician Salt to resurrect Prince Albert after his death. The spell succeeded, but in addition to reviving Prince Albert it also brought back "everything else that had ever been dead besides" (issue 8, p. 10). The Curse's origin thus proves not an instance of the colonized writing back to the Empire as speculated by Bowes's mother, but nonetheless still represents an instance of the Empire being punished for hubris and overreaching: seeking to exert dominion over life and death, and consequently suffering horrible consequences. The way the narrative connects zombie etiology to Prince Albert's death, proximate to the rise of germ theory and rapid imperial expansion between the 1870s and 1900, suggests that the imperial—in addition to the "scientific"—crimes of the Victorian era have come back to haunt the Edwardian period.[4] Thus analogies between the zombies and the colonized are thematically potent, generating resonances between imperial and scientific hubris. Abnett and Culbard flirt briefly with the theme of scientists playing God when a priest, speaking to Suttle, argues that the Restless plague must be God's plan: "Because if it was not, then it was the work of man, and that is a crime beyond imagination" (issue 7, p. 14). Whereas Mary Shelley's *Frankenstein* posits the hubris of the scientist meddling with life to create a human being, *The New Deadwardians* depicts all life being put at risk to save one royal life, Prince Albert's. Whereas *Frankenstein* discusses science's potential to create life from inanimate material, zombie narratives create medical interventions as weapons and viruses, as in the film *28 Days Later* (Danny Boyle 2003), although sometimes the pathogen can develop in the wild strains as in Max Brooks's novel *World War Z* (2006) (adapted into a film in 2013).

The New Deadwardians is less interested in questions of forbidden knowledge than in ones of how such knowledge, once acquired, is commodified. Who is granted or denied access to it and what are the consequences of this access or denial? This focus is seen most explicitly in the comic's depiction of how the Cure is harnessed and controlled by those in power. Class division is predicated on access, or lack thereof, to this asset. Access or lack thereof also dictates whether one becomes a vampire, a zombie, or zombie food. In exploring this terrain, Abnett and Culbard generate resonances between past and present and question the role of and access to medicalization in our own era, evoking controversial healthcare discourses such as Obamacare and the role of the pharmaceutical industry.

"All Equally Dead": Signifiers of the Curse and Symptoms of the Cure

While they are never actually labeled zombies, the Restless are clearly zombie creatures: they have an appetite for human flesh; appear to be dead, with sickly green complexions and decomposing features; and are most efficiently dispatched via bullet to the head. These creatures occupy the outskirts of Zone B, the poor and working-class district of London, fenced off from its inhabitants, the Bright, and kept at considerable distance from the Young inhabiting the upscale Zone A. Culbard's art frequently depicts the creatures gathered in hordes at barricades and fences, segregated from humankind by man-made structures (issue 1, p. 10; issue 2, p. 12; issue 3, pp. 5–6). As in other popular zombie texts, the dead in *The New Deadwardians* wait by these structures ravenous for what lies on the other side: "The Restless gather thick at the barrier fence, drawn by the scent of life. Somehow they can still smell it over the odor of death they exude" (issue 3, p. 3).

In *The New Deadwardians*, however, it is not only humans who lie on the other side of the partition. It is also home to the Young, who came about through a substance designed to defeat the Restless. Suttle reflects, "When the stratagem of warfare didn't stop the Restless, the ruling classes took the Cure instead. Allowing ourselves to become technically dead rendered us invisible to the Cursed. It was superlative pragmatism . . . We chose to become Young because it made us dead enough to fool the fully undead. It was the only thing we cared about. We hadn't the least idea what else it might do to us" (issue 2, pp. 6–7). The juxtaposition of this text with a close-up image of a zombie face—decaying, eyes aglow, with maggots in its gaping mouth—highlights the gravity of the threat that must be eliminated, namely, the diseased ghoul, but with the caveat "We hadn't the least idea what else it might do to us" foreshadowing the equivalent monstrosity that befalls those who take the Cure. Of his own medicating via the Cure, Suttle recalls, "I was on a week's leave in London. The Cure had been developed. A new weapon. They wanted all officers to take it. They explained it would proof us against the Restless. It didn't occur to me to argue. I just took it" (issue 4, p. 18).

The use of the name "the Cure" is illuminating and layered: as a descriptor it is medicinal but also finite, sweeping, hubristic, and presumptive; it carries connotations not only of healing elixirs but of dominant cultures throughout different eras forcing solutions on perceived threats of social difference (e.g., homosexuality, minorities, and communism). Its function as both a medicinal substance and military stratagem—"a new weapon"— highlights its dual status as savior and threat, and such negative connotations are fitting given the dominant culture's use and control of the Cure.

The New Deadwardians deliberately obscures the precise nature of the Cure, as well as its origin, development, and manufacture. However, its administration is visually depicted as similar to a blood transfusion (issue 1, p. 11; issue 4, p. 18), a process that, at the time of the comic's main action, the early 1900s, was increasingly commonplace. The deliberate vagueness about the Cure's ingredients and how it works enable readers to generate their own associations between it and other medical practices. For example, the fact that the Young must regularly take the Cure—early in the story Suttle notes that he is "overdue" (issue 1, p. 9)—generates a number of potential correspondences: those who read it as a blood transfusion of sorts might identify in this a further link to vampirism; others may identify links to vaccination, given that vaccination requires boosters; and others may identify aspects of twentieth-century antibiotic culture in the Cure, whereby dependency on drugs weakens the immune systems and curtails the potential to develop natural immunity. The investigators wonder if the Cure is failing after finding a dead member of the Young, something that should be medically impossible (issue 2, p. 5), a sentiment that echoes fears of antibiotic resistance in the twenty-first century and the reemergence of health problems deemed solved for a century. Hence the Cure provides a blank canvas on which readers can project a number of medical equivalents. By not tethering their critique too explicitly to any particular medical substance, practice, or custom, Abnett and Culbard ensure the focus is on the misuse of such resources predicated on wealth and access rather than the resources themselves. This is consistent with other zombie narratives whose focus is generally on the subsequent social formations rather than the intricacies of causes and solutions.

The Cure is also noteworthy as a defective substance, however. On the surface it fulfilled its primary function, rendering the Young invisible to the Restless and enabling them to approach undetected for combat. However, its repercussions prove multiple. The Young are never explicitly labeled vampires, but their symptoms evoke many of the defining characteristics of vampirism. While the Young can walk around in sunlight, they must wear zinc paste and hats to do so; they do not age and cannot die of natural causes, and typically can only be killed via "impalement of the heart, decapitation, incineration" (issue 1, p. 20); they grow fangs and must file their teeth back for the sake of decorum; and animals keep their distance. Suttle also recognizes fundamental similarities between his Young brethren and the Restless, noting that "we are so alike in our lifeless lives. I am eternal and sentient. They are enduring and mindless. But otherwise we are all equally dead" (issue 3, p. 6). The imagery accompanying this text—Suttle staring directly into a zombie's eyes through the bars of a fence, with Suttle on the left of the panel and the zombie on the right, evoking a mirror image—highlights this central contradiction. On the one hand, Suttle and the Restless are segregated by fencing and are distinguished from one another aesthetically, but, on the other hand, the zombie holds a mirror up to Suttle and his ilk, emphasizing their fundamental similarities. This reinforces the idea that abuse of medical resources negatively affects both those with access and those without, albeit in different ways.

The New Deadwardians problematizes the superficial binary of zombification as disease and Cure as cure. The Cure does not really "cure" the contagion—the zombie population is never eliminated and infection continues—and indeed proves more a curse. While the Young are invulnerable to the Restless, Abnett and Culbard dramatize the loss, both personal and psychical, that results from taking this substance, most notably a loss of human appetites and passion for life itself, as epitomized by Suttle. Like medications such as chemotherapy and some hepatitis treatments, this cure for zombiism is a type of disease and results in a lifetime of diminished bodily capacity.

One key difference between the Young and the Restless is that while the Restless have unquenchable appetites, most Young do not. Suttle laments that "the worst part of being Young . . . is a lack of human appetite. For food, for drink, for love, for life" (issue 4, p. 5). Elsewhere he mourns the erosion of his sexual desire, commenting, "Before I took the Cure, I was a healthy young man. I had desires. Passions. I had what I believe is known as a libido" (issue 3, p. 11). The flashback panel depicting Suttle taking the Cure emphasizes his sacrifice. From a high angle Suttle is shown lying shirtless, arms extended out in a crucifixion pose, with a priest holding a bible to his left and doctors surrounding him, supervising a blood transfusion (issue 4, p. 18). On the one hand this image echoes portraits and depictions of Christ on the cross, conjuring images of martyrdom and self-sacrifice, but on the other hand it evokes images of lethal injection of convicts, symbolically recasting the Cure as a death sentence. The connection between medical cure and religious salvation, and the loss inherent in both, reminds us that the shift from mythical/religious-based monstrosity to medico-scientific monstrosity is a real concern. We see this reflected in the recent tendency for popular culture to replace mythical or religious causes of monstrous metamorphosis with disease- and infection-based ones, for example, in zombie texts such as *28 Days Later* or vampire ones such as *The Strain* (novel 2009; television 2014–). To place the causes of monstrosity in medico-scientific landscapes brings the concerns into the realm of the everyday for the audience, slotting neatly into a media landscape saturated with alarmist narratives of SARS, swine flu, and Ebola. Such narratives raise questions about religious salvation, and *The New Deadwardians* additionally questions religion's role in a world without death.

The visual depiction of Suttle accentuates this theme of living death: he is pale, his posture awkward and stiff, his complexion and manner lethargic and grim: arguably he is the dreariest protagonist ever to headline a series from the Vertigo label. However, while Suttle is stiff and dispassionate (at least until rediscovering reserves of passion later in the series), other members of the Young develop alternative and sometimes transgressive passions, such as the urge to bite and drink blood: the prostitute Sapphire informs Suttle that "the Cure takes some right funny. Gives them tendencies. Urges they cannot control. Urges to bite and drink" (issue 3, p. 13). Ultimately, whether passionless or plagued by aberrant passions distorted into vampiric fetish, the paradox of the Cure is that "the very point of living [i.e., love, emotion] disappears at the precise moment that you're given an endless slice of lifetime to use up" (issue 5, p. 15). A medicine created to preserve humanity ultimately erodes or perverts the very humanity it is meant to save, drawing attention to the misuse of medical knowledge and substances and suggesting that such misuse ultimately damages those who benefit as well as those denied access.

Zone B: What Became of the Working Class?

The Young clearly occupy the upper class, mobile middle class, and positions of authority in the comic's class framework, with the Restless as the abject on society's fringes. This conflation of aristocracy with vampirism is a popular fictional trope, dating at least to Bram Stoker's *Dracula* (1897), and the conflation of zombies with lower classes is similarly long-standing. The Bright, meanwhile, occupy the working class, wedged between the Young and the Restless, possessing their lives and faculties but without luxuries or access to symbols of status. In this respect, while human, the Bright are aligned with zombies in their class status: a scene featuring an altercation between Suttle and labor union protesters, for example, resembles images elsewhere in the book of zombies attacking (issue 6, pp. 19–20; issue 7, p. 1). The segregation of the Bright into a special zone, much as the Restless are segregated, accentuates the point about equitable access to medical assets, highlighting the extent to which where one lives can be the biggest determinant of health and building on the centuries-old view of East London as contaminated.

The geography of London is keenly felt throughout. The Young occupy Zone A, the West End; the Bright occupy Zone B, the East End; and the Restless predominantly cluster around this second zone. The image of the entry point to Zone B, ostensibly a gateway and scaffold, presents a mess of structures and bars and fences, reinforcing the visual motif of boundaries and barricades discussed previously that runs throughout the book as well as evoking a Foucauldian politics of segregation and compartmentalization (issue 3, p. 1). This vision of the East End of London as diseased, as something to be segregated, and the West End as healthy goes back as far as the late Victorian era, and perhaps earlier, according to Paul Newland (2008). The rise of health concerns in the Victorian era saw the medical establishment, supported by the health surveillance measures, exacerbate the division between the East and West sides of the city. For Newland, the depiction of the East End is politically motivated and is a space in which "anxieties" about English identity are, in effect, quarantined (24), a motif mirrored in *The New Deadwardians* in its literal quarantining of the Bright and the Restless who threaten "proper" English identity—that is, the dominant upper and middle-class culture.

Newland draws on Elizabeth Grosz's work to elucidate how London has been understood through metaphors of the human body. Grosz (1998, 43) writes, "The city is made and made over into the simulacrum of the body, and the body, in its turn, is transformed, 'citified,' urbanized as a distinctively metropolitan body." However, the capacity for disease to significantly shape both bodily and political identity is not purely symbolic. For Priscilla Wald (2008, 82), "contagion in general was a fact of, as well as a metaphor for, life in the crowded conditions of urban spaces. Tenements of immigrants and migrants offered the most visible representation of the excesses of industrialization and of the limits of assimilation." This view is mirrored in the comic's depiction of infection and zombies teeming within the city limit and especially its depiction of the zombie hordes gathered outside the zones, rabid to penetrate the borders keeping them out. This also corresponds to images and narratives of outnumbered colonists at the margins of the Empire protecting, in their view, a modicum of civility against the threat of the invading, and infecting, hordes.

For Newland, the East End is conceived and consistently represented as the "sick, diseased and cancerous part of the body of the city" (2008, 16), and he points out that these images are so dominant that during the city's bid for the 2012 Olympic Games "discourses of bodily development and renewal" emerged, highlighting the inherent connections between cities and the bodies that inhabit them (15). Newland draws on example after example to show the conflation of East End London with bodily infection, and *The New Deadwardians* taps into these metaphors with its central drama of infected bodies requiring containment or elimination.

This depiction of the East End as diseased is evident in the comic's visual style. Patricia Mulvihill's color palette is subdued, deploying predominantly grays, mustards, and browns, colors associated with illness and decay. However, red is used strategically throughout for dramatic as well as thematic effect. The first major splashes of red appear in the opening pages, where Suttle wakes up to discover his housekeeper being devoured by a zombie, with a pool of blood spilling from her corpse (issue 1, p. 3). Suttle wears a red dressing gown in this scene, which contrasts with the red of the housekeeper's blood and creates an immediate visual association between the two different versions of the undead, foreshadowing Suttle's own observations about their inherent similarities later in the narrative. The fact that the first victim is Suttle's housekeeper also reinforces the class themes: Suttle, holding a civil service post, represents the upwardly mobile middle class but also, as son of a dowager-like persona, embodies aristocracy as well. The association of red with zombiism and vampirism is reinforced elsewhere, with the color used primarily for blood and zombie gore, on the one hand, and for soldiers' uniforms—the wardrobe of the militaristic Young—on the other (issue 2, p. 6; issue 4, p. 19). Slaughtering colonizers and the slaughtered colonized are thus visually linked.

Underscoring the importance of location and geography throughout is a map of London, tinted red, which separates issues in the trade paperback. The use of red here, in addition to reinforcing the links between geography and other motifs coded red, also reinforces the state of continuing insecurity within the city (red being the color most commonly used to signify danger). In "The Victorian Social Body and Urban Cartography," Pamela Gilbert (2002, 13) identifies the cholera outbreak as the impetus for medical mapping as a public health practice, used to deploy resources in a time of crisis; however, she also points out that the result is "the spatialized understanding of social problems." Abnett and Culbard's map evokes John Snow's contemporaneous cholera maps, detailing outbreaks and infection events, that were instrumental in epidemiologically based decision making, such as the closure of the Broad Street water pump in 1854 (Gilbert 2002, 18–19).

Furthermore, on colonial maps red can signify, if unintentionally, the death of indigenous populations to shore up territorial and financial wealth, and here the bloody map signifies the death and destruction of lower-class lives in service of upper-class health and well-being. Gilbert (2008, 7) writes that the growing threat of cholera in the Victorian era served as a "prime actor" linking public health and national identity in England and its Empire. According to her, "the dramatic eruption of an alien and frightening epidemic during conditions of reform agitation provided unique practical and narrative opportunities" (8). So, too, does the eruption of the Restless curse in *The New Deadwardians* prove a catalyst for "practical and narrative opportunities," albeit of a less benevolent and more sinister kind, namely, the use of the Cure to maintain dominant class structures.

While the spread of disease does not distinguish by class in *The New Deadwardians*, class initiates the disease and informs the counterresponse. As the critic William Kulesa observes (2012), "This is a story of people recovering from an event that fundamentally changed their reality, and [they] are determined to adhere to the old forms as much as possible." The Bright are not granted access to the Cure and are vulnerable to the Restless due to their visibility (not to mention proximity) and consequently exposed to death by zombie attack and death by zombie infection, which would transform them into the living dead.

Despite its evident drawbacks, those in power who benefit most from its existence advocate for the Cure. These are class assignations pushed to their extremes. Suttle's superior Carstairs provides a typically militaristic, biopolitical justification for the Cure: "We took the bloody Cure for the good of the Empire. . . . No one wanted to. No one liked it. Bloody Restless were eating us alive. We got on with it to keep this country together. For king and country" (issue 2, pp. 5–6). The use of the word "took" here and elsewhere when describing the Cure can be read in multiple ways. On the one hand, when Suttle talks of having "took" the Cure, with "took" emphasized in bold (issue 4, p. 18), the connotation is that he is submitting to it, whereas when other military and upper classes speak of having "took" the Cure, as above, it carries a connotation of seizing and not sharing. Indeed, the Cure is both a military initiative and a product of the Victorian/Edwardian era: hence, powerful men decide access. Hinchcliffe's activist daughter Celia links the control of the Cure's distribution by men to the gender inequalities of the era, stating, "Women's suffrage will not advance until we are granted equality in all things, including the right to determine our own immortality" (issue 5, p. 9). One woman who takes the Cure is Suttle's maid, who at the start of the series is bitten by one of the Restless. Suttle takes his maid to receive the Cure, and while an instance of a lower-class citizen being granted this boon, it is anomalous and enabled only through the intervention of her master.

Suttle's remark that the Cure renders the Young "dead enough to fool the fully undead" (issue 2, pp. 6–7) is also indicative of the tactical thinking, ulterior motives, and subterfuge inherent in the Cure. This, ultimately, is the key thematic preoccupation of the series: the Cure, whatever its shortcomings, is a medical asset, one that empowers those who control it to remain the dominant power in society, in much the same way that access to and control of any powerful resource dictates leadership and power. Abnett and Culbard critique such exploitation of medications and tools created for the betterment of humankind. The Cure was created as a means of defeating the Restless hordes fifty years past; therefore, it was developed to benefit humanity, yet access to it has been restricted largely to the ruling class and authorities. The Cure, and by extension medicine, become social capital, and the series contends that the misuse of this resource is universally detrimental. Those with access live longer and exert dominion over the Empire but have lost their humanity in fundamental ways and—perhaps through circuitous, symbolic karma—are rendered passionless, impotent, or psychosexually perverse.

The comic's horror tropes and period setting are important for conveying these ideas. The use of zombies and vampires provides recognizable metaphors and illuminates parallels to the contemporary United States. Although written by a British author and located in Edwardian London, the series was published by an American imprint—Vertigo, a division of DC Comics—and speaks predominantly to the exploitation and inequitable dissemination of medical knowledge and access by world superpowers, of which the modern United States is the primary contemporary example. According to de Groot (2009), historical fiction frequently concerns the rise of the nation-state and is used as a way of making sense of national identity in ways more observable from the safety of the present. Moreover, Bill Ashcroft, Gareth Griffiths, and Helen Tiffin (1989, 7) argue that "Britain, like the other dominant colonial powers of the nineteenth century, has been relegated to a relatively minor place in international affairs. Nonetheless, through the literary canon, the body of British texts which all too frequently still acts as a touchstone of taste and value . . . the weight of antiquity continues to dominate cultural production in much of the post-colonial world." In short, the vocabulary of contemporary imperialism and colonialism— medical, geographical, and otherwise—is the vocabulary established by Britain and its literary canon, and Edwardian London provides a fitting vehicle for Abnett and Culbard's critique of our contemporary misuse of knowledge and power.

While the crises depicted in *The New Deadwardians* are obviously inflated due to the comic's horror content, their real-world equivalents are compelling and pertinent. The lack of access to the Cure for middle- and lower-class citizens is reflected in our own economics of healthcare: at the time of this writing, forty-four million people in the United States do not possess any health insurance and thirty-eight million possess health insurance that is inadequate, and these are predominantly working-class citizens (PBS 2014). Such inequalities are also reflected on a global scale: for example, bodies such as Médecins Sans Frontières have criticized the West for its slowness to act in response to the 2014 West African Ebola outbreak, arguing that it was not until the Ebola virus began affecting Western citizens that major world powers chose to intervene with research, medical, and financial aid (O'Carroll 2014). Much as these sorts of injustices lead to social unrest in *The New Deadwardians*, so, too, do they in reality: indeed, the year prior to the publication of *The New Deadwardians* saw the emergence of the

Occupy movement across the United States. While the balance of power and distribution of access to medical resources remains largely intact at narrative's end, much as the balance of power remains so in reality, Abnett and Culbard's central thesis is clear: when resources are not shared, the Cure kills us all. Moreover, by utilizing a historical setting that parallels the contemporary moment, along with graphic storytelling and recognizable horror archetypes with built-in class assignations, these creators harness the simultaneous otherness and familiarity of the past to address these topical concerns around medical ethics and equity.

NOTES

1. The use of the terms "Young" and "Restless" jokingly evokes the CBS soap opera series *The Young and the Restless* (1973–), which itself originated as a chronicle of families from opposing classes.
2. Such fears and Othering permeate narratives of illness and epidemic; as Wald (2008, 8) notes, racist attitudes underpinned reporting and public perception of SARS.
3. For a reading of how the physician-author Arthur Conan Doyle negotiates this notion, see Yumna Siddiqi's (2006) "The Cesspool of Empire: Sherlock Holmes and the Return of the Repressed."
4. This included British competition for new territories in Africa, resulting in conflicts such as the Boer Wars, and the crowning of Queen Victoria as the empress of India in 1877. In medical terms, we can also link this to the complicity of British tropical medicine in the country's imperial conquests.

REFERENCES

Abnett, Dan, and I. N. J. Culbard. 2013. *The New Deadwardians*. Trade paperback. New York: Vertigo, DC Comics.

Anderson, Warwick. 1995. "Excremental Colonialism: Public Health and the Poetics of Pollution." *Critical Inquiry* 21 (3): 640–69.

Ashcroft, Bill, Gareth Griffiths, and Helen Tiffin. 1989. *The Empire Writes Back: Theory and Practice in Post-colonial Literatures*. London: Routledge.

Bashford, Alison. 2000. "Is White Australia Possible? Race, Colonialism, and Tropical Medicine." *Ethnic and Racial Studies* 23 (2): 248–71.

Conrad, Peter. 2008. *The Medicalization of Society: On the Transformation of Human Conditions into Treatable Disorders*. Baltimore: Johns Hopkins University Press.

De Groot, Jerome. 2009. *The Historical Novel*. London: Routledge.

Gilbert, Pamela. 2002. "The Victorian Social Body and Urban Cartography." In *Imagined Londons*, edited by Pamela Gilbert, 11–30. Albany: State University of New York Press.

———. 2004. "Mapping and Social Space in Nineteenth-Century England." In *Mapping the Victorian Social Body*, edited by Pamela Gilbert, 3–26. Albany: State University of New York Press.

———. 2008. *Cholera and Nation: Doctoring the Social Body in Victorian England*. Albany: State University of New York Press.

Grosz, Elizabeth. 1998. "Bodies-Cities." In *Places through the Body*, edited by Heidi Nast and Steve Pile, 42–51. London: Routledge.

Inguanzo, Ozzy. 2014. *Zombies on Film: The Definitive Story of Undead Cinema*. New York: Universe.

Kulesa, William. 2012. "*The New Deadwardians* Is a Murder Mystery Layered with Social Psychology of Class." *Jersey Journal*, April 12. http://www.nj.com/jjournal-news/index.ssf/2012/04/the_new_deadwardians_is_a_murd.html.

Newland, Paul. 2008. *The Cultural Construction of London's East End: Urban Iconography, Modernity, and the Spatialisation of Englishness*. New York: Rodopi.

O'Carroll, Lisa. 2014. "World's Ebola Response Slow, Patchy, and Inadequate, Médecins sans Frontières Says." *The Guardian*, December 3. http://www.theguardian.com/global-development/2014/dec/02/ebola-medecins-sans-frontieres-west-africa.

PBS. 2014. "Healthcare Crisis: Who's at Risk." http://www.pbs.org/healthcarecrisis.

Philip, John. 1828. *Researches in South Africa Illustrating the Civil, Moral, and Religious Condition of the Native Tribes, etc.* London: James Duncan. https://archive.org/stream/researchesinsou00philgoog/researchesinsou00philgoog_djvu.txt.

Roberts, Timothy. 2006. "Dead Ends: The Spectre of Elitism in the Zombie Film." *Philament* 9 (December): 1–14.

Round, Julia. 2014. *Gothic in Comics and Graphic Novels: A Critical Approach*. Jefferson, NC: McFarland.

Siddiqi, Yumna. 2006. "The Cesspool of Empire: Sherlock Holmes and Return of the Repressed." *Victorian Literature and Culture* 34 (1): 233–47.

Wald, Priscilla. 2008. *Contagious: Cultures, Carriers, and the Outbreak Narrative*. Durham, NC: Duke University Press.

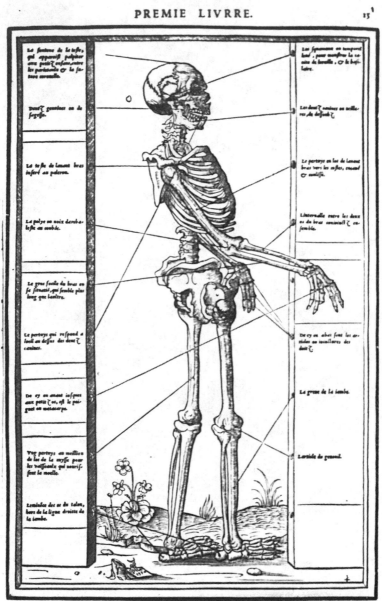

Le fontaine de la teste, qui apparoist palpiter aux petis enfans, entre les parietaux & la suture coronale.

Deux gouttieres ou de sagesse.

La teste de l'vn des bras inseré en paleron.

La polye ou noix derrabelesse en nœbôe.

Le gros fosille du bras en se fermant, qui semble plus long que l'autre.

Le portoys qui respond a l'oeil au dessus des deux canines.

De cy en amont iusques aux petis os, est le paiquet en metacarpe.

Vne portoys ou moelle de los de la cuisse pour les vaisseaux qui nourrissent la moelle.

La miniere des os du talon, hors de la ligne droitte de la iambe.

Les fignament ou temporal bas, pour monstrer la cavité de l'oreille, & le basilaire.

Les deux canines ou veilleros, au dessous.

Le portoys ou los de l'vn des bras vers les costes, creusé & oualissé.

L'interualle entre les deux os du bras comiault ensemble.

De cy en abas sont les articles ou iauailleres des dois.

Le gros de la iambe.

L'article du genoül.

PART 2: READING THE ZOMBIE METAPHOR

4.

THE WALKING MED

Zombies, Comics, and Medical Education

Michael Green, Daniel George, and Darryl Wilkinson

Introduction

This is an essay about zombies, comics, and medical education, three nouns that do not typically appear in a single sentence. When approached to write this chapter, I (Michael Green) initially responded, "But I don't know anything about zombies! I have never seen a zombie movie or read a zombie comic book, and I am not a fan of zombie literature. As an internist and bioethicist, I have no qualifications to write the chapter!" But after educating myself and reflecting on the topic, I soon realized that many of the tropes appearing in zombie literature (e.g., alienation, dehumanization, and survival) echo the themes I had been seeing in the comics that my fourth-year medical students were creating for a course I teach on comics and medicine. I discussed this with my colleague Danny George, an anthropologist and zombie enthusiast, and with Danny's friend Darryl Wilkinson, an archaeologist by training and a zombiephile by passion. The three of us came together to write this essay. So, what happens when an internist, an anthropologist, and an archaeologist walk into a bar . . . or, in this case, write about zombies, comics, and medical education? What follows is the fruit of our labor.

Zombies, Popular Culture, and Medicine

These days, zombies are everywhere. Once a fringe figure, the zombie is now the dominant strain of the undead within popular culture. The last fifteen years in particular have seen something of an explosion in popular interest in zombies across virtually all media—including television, cinema, graphic and traditional novels, the Internet, and computer games (Drezner 2011).

Academics and researchers—never outside of popular culture—have also been drawn into the modern zombie craze. Zombies and their theoretical conceivability are used as a mainstay for thought experiments in philosophy, resulting in heated debates on the material basis of consciousness,[1] and scholars in the fields of cultural studies, sociology, and anthropology have explored the zombie as a critical metaphor for describing the effects of global capitalism and mass consumption on human lives and society.[2]

Professionals and academics working in the medical fields seem no less enamored with the zombie concept. In 2011 the US Centers for Disease Control and Prevention made international headlines when it published a blog post (and later a full-length digital graphic novel) on how to survive a zombie apocalypse—a deliberate attempt to publicize disaster preparedness strategies by playing on the popularity of zombies (Sherryl Vint explores this text in her chapter in this volume; see also Silver et al. 2011). Similarly, in an article on popular perceptions of individuals with dementia, Susan M. Behuniak (2011) critically considered the portrayal of Alzheimer's patients as the "living dead,"[3] showing the potentially harmful and dehumanizing effects of the zombie allegory in certain medical contexts.

As an object of horror, loathing, and fascination, the zombie functions as a powerful and resonant metaphor for a variety of present-day fears and worries, reflecting subliminal concerns that might otherwise be difficult to articulate via common discourse. In this chapter we are concerned with zombie tropes within medical circles, but in contexts that are distinct from those considered by other scholars. Although related to analyses such as Behuniak's (2011), our focus is on the use of zombie metaphors as applied to medical trainees rather than patients. In particular, we focus on how the zombie metaphor plays out in the minds of medical students—individuals who are undergoing formative professionalization experiences at the beginning stages of their careers. Like other contributors to this volume, we are interested in exploring the representation of zombies in graphic narratives (or comics). However, the materials that directly concern us are not those published accounts that are created for mass circulation, like *Marvel Zombies* (2005–6) or *The Walking Dead* (2003–). Instead, they are the images and narratives produced by six cohorts of medical students who created comics as part of their coursework in medical school. These comics are personal, semiprivate reflections addressing the challenges of medical education, and they are mainly intended for an audience of peers and instructors.

By exploring comics in this very specific biomedical context, we will reference the wider study of zombie metaphors in modern culture. But why would zombie themes resonate with medical students at all? Upon review of six years of student comics, we found that zombie tropes appear throughout these works, raising several questions that serve as a concise introduction to the issues we wish to address in this essay: What is it about the experience of medical professionalization and the culture of medicine that seems apt to being expressed through the use of zombie metaphors? Does creating comics free students to express themselves in ways that would be more difficult using other mediums? What does the embrace of zombie tropes reveal about the meaning of medical school to students? Given that zombification is ostensibly a "negative thing," should the medical students' use of this expressive form give us pause when thinking about how medical education is presently structured?

Metaphors have power because using the nonliteral helps us express and explore our everyday experiences. We doubt medical students genuinely fear that viral contamination will turn them into actual zombies. Instead, zombie fiction and the tropes it deploys are in some sense "good to think with" because they capture something about existing fears and anxieties without having to convey them in purely realistic or literal terms. If zombies and zombification encapsulate something of the experience of medical students as they learn to become physicians, then we should pay attention to such metaphors, consider what aspects of students' experiences are being expressed through them, and think deeply about what medical educators can do to push back against the culture of medicine that is producing such anxieties in its trainees.

A Course on Comics and Medicine for Medical Students

At this point, one might wonder about the origins of this discussion on zombies and comics in medical education. After all, medical schools are typically understood to be serious training environments that would not generally afford opportunities to explore depictions of zombies or other fantastical creatures. That said, for the past six years, one of us (Michael Green) has been teaching "Comics and Medicine," a course for fourth-year medical students at Penn State College of Medicine. This is one offering among many humanities "selectives" in which students are required to enroll during their final year of medical school.

For the course, students read medically themed comics and create their own original comic, drawn from a formative experience during their training. This provides opportunities not only for critical analysis but also for personal reflection and creative expression. Details regarding the rationale and logistics of this course have been described elsewhere (Green 2013, 2015), so here we focus on the comics that students create. In broad terms, students are asked to produce an original story about a memorable experience from medical school using words and images. Guidance and mentoring are provided, and the course is structured as a seminar/workshop with ample opportunities for reflection and discussion about students' creative work.

The course lasts for four weeks and meets for two and a half hours, twice per week. Since it takes place during the final year of medical school, students have already accumulated some clinical experience and have made decisions about the areas of medicine in which they will specialize. Such factors greatly influence students' responses to the first class assignment, which involves reacting to open-ended writing prompts[4] about formative experiences from school, such as:

- One thing about being a medical student that my family doesn't understand is . . .
- My proudest moment as a medical student was . . .
- I was really impressed with a colleague when s/he . . .
- One of the most troubling things I experienced as a medical student was . . .
- It was especially hard for me to deal with my patient when s/he . . .

After committing their responses to paper, students pair up to share their thoughts and experiences—an activity that generates animated discussion. Their homework assignment is to reflect further and begin to shape one or more of these experiences into a story that contains a beginning, middle, and end. Students are instructed that the story should: (1) describe an interesting experience from medical school; (2) reveal something about a formative experience; (3) tell something about the medical school culture; and (4) be worth sharing with others. During subsequent sessions, students discuss these stories and begin to transform one of them into a comic. At the same time, students read a variety of medically themed graphic narratives, Skype with authors, and practice their drawing and creative-writing skills.

Given the open-ended nature of the writing prompts, it is not surprising that the stories students tell are quite varied. Some focus on an uplifting incident, such as the student heroically helping a patient through a medical crisis, while others present darker views of the medical school experience, reflecting students' fears and worries about who they are, how they have changed, and who they may become in the future. The use of the comics medium frees students to express themselves both visually and metaphorically. In so doing, they depict not only the explicit lessons taught via lectures and seminars but also the "hidden curriculum" of medical school—the norms, values, and beliefs learned from direct observation and exposure to clinical environments that can undermine the formal classroom messages (Hafferty 1998).

Unlike most courses in medical school that aim to teach detailed information or technical skills to developing professionals, the "Comics and Medicine" course sparks students to look at how the past four years have imprinted on their professional and personal development—especially in terms of how it has shaped them as practitioners and, ultimately, as people. For many students, this is the first time during medical school they have a chance to slow down, step back, and reflect on the totality of their medical training thus far. That zombies are part of that reflection is intriguing.

It Is Not About the Zombies

The idea of zombies, of course, predates modern biomedical medical education. Originally a creature from Haitian folklore, a *zombi* was a human revenant enslaved to the will of the sorcerer who had magically reanimated him or her. It was not, however, until the 1932 release of the first motion picture on the topic (*White Zombie*, starring Bela Lugosi and directed by Victor Halperin) that the zombie concept began to circulate widely beyond its Caribbean origins and achieve its present status as a staple of global popular fiction. Although other manifestations of the undead such as ghosts, vampires, and mummies may have been more commonplace throughout most of the twentieth century, in recent decades zombies have been rapidly catching up, and medical students—like others in contemporary American life—seem drawn to zombie references as they reflect on their own recent experiences.

Even so, one of the great ironies about the proliferation of zombies in popular culture and literature is that these stories are not ultimately about zombies. Rather, zombies are used as backdrops for story lines about survivors and the relationships that emerge in response to apocalyptic disasters. George Romero (2014), writer and director of numerous zombie films including the landmark *Night of the Living Dead* (1968), explained that "the zombies are just sort of out there. They could be a hurricane or a typhoon or anything. They're the disaster that everyone is facing. But my stories are more about the humans."

In zombified worlds, questions inevitably arise about how people react when confronted by danger: Do they band together, or is everyone out for him- or herself? Do people help the least advantaged, or is it survival of the fittest? How do people cope with stress—calmly or with panic? How are power relationships negotiated—do the smartest become leaders, or do the strong and ruthless take over? In other words, the zombie apocalypse provides context for exploring what it means to be human (and also humane) in the face of deep adversity. In that case, perhaps the zombies are a kind of reminder of the always-present potential to lose one's humanity as a response to strife—simultaneously the force of disaster and a cautionary tale.

Although these questions are particularly relevant to the zombie oeuvre, they also resonate with the stories created by medical students. And, while it would be an exaggeration to describe the working conditions of a hospital and the experiences of medical students as equivalent to surviving a zombie apocalypse, medical school training nevertheless occurs in an environment infamous for high pressure, stress, and uncertainty. Thus, in such environments, it is instructive to see how students respond and react to the conditions in which they find themselves. As with the heterogeneity of responses in zombie literature, the medical trainees react in diverse ways.

So what do medical students have in common with zombies (or with human survivors)? In the remainder of this essay we will explore students' use of zombie metaphors to describe some of the dehumanizing aspects of their medical school experiences.

Zombie Metaphors and Medical Education

Isolation and Loneliness

Perhaps the best place to start is by setting the scene. A common and recurring theme in zombie fiction is the experience of sheer isolation and loneli-

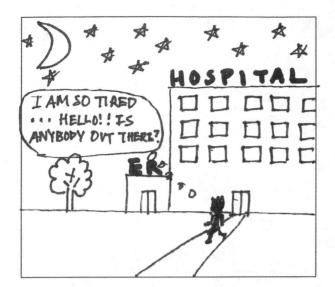

ness. Cinematographically, this often leads to images of the protagonist wandering through an empty landscape, now devoid of (living) people— something often found in apocalyptic fiction in general. A typical example of this would be the opening sequences of the movie *28 Days Later* (Danny Boyle 2003), as well as the first episode of the television show *The Walking Dead* (2010–), in which the main character awakens in an abandoned hospital, initially unaware that the zombie apocalypse has occurred while he lay comatose.

A similar sense of alienation while moving within a lifeless, empty space is found in the graphic narratives produced by some of the medical students in the "Comics and Medicine" course. For instance, in the comic produced by Kie Lee (2010), the landscape around the hospital where he works is characterized by barren buildings lacking any other people. In one section, Lee depicts the student (himself) stepping out into the empty landscape around the hospital during the unsociable hours required by his clinical rotation and forlornly asking, "Is anybody out there?"

Lee is quite explicit about his reference to zombie tropes elsewhere in his narrative; in one section he openly states, "I felt like a zombie," and shows himself as a zombified individual, with both his arms held horizontal in the classic zombie pose.

In the case of Lee's work in particular, the ways in which solitude is expressed, in both the text and the depiction of landscapes, can be readily understood as influenced by zombie fiction. His experience of solitude is

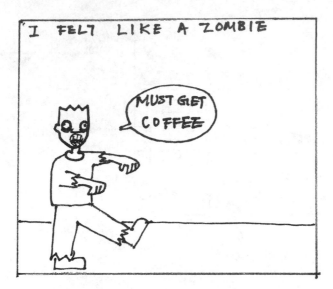

4.2 From Kie Lee, "My First Big Case" (2010).

intimately tied to the hours during which medical students are required to work (it is clearly night when he arrives for his shift and again when he leaves at its conclusion). The hyperbolic comparison here lies between the postapocalyptic landscapes of fiction and the medical student's experience of a sleep-deprived world where one's work schedule rarely allows access to daylight. The use of zombie metaphors in Lee's comic is a powerful reminder of the challenges medical students face in trying to sustain a "normal" life during medical school, suggesting that disruptive rhythms and unusual daily routines are a particularly difficult aspect of medical education.

Mindless Consumption

For many scholars of popular culture, the most fundamental theme of zombie fiction is its metaphorical depiction—and critique—of the consumer society of the late twentieth and early twenty-first centuries. The most widely cited example of this is George Romero's film *Dawn of the Dead* (1978), which revolves around a group of survivors who occupy a shopping mall as a refuge from the zombie horde and delight in the unfettered consumption of the various goods the mall offers them. As aptly put by the scholar Kyle Bishop (2010, 234), "By setting the bulk of the action in a shopping mall, Romero consciously draws the audience's attention toward the relationship between zombies and consumerism. The insatiable need to purchase, own, and consume has become so deeply ingrained in twentieth-

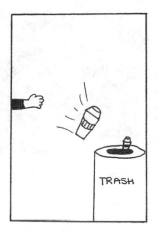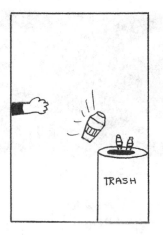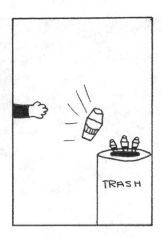

4.3 From Christian Squillante, untitled (2009).

century Americans that their reanimated corpses are relentlessly driven by the same instincts and needs."

Given the tendency of scholars to read the contemporary popularity of the zombie as, fundamentally, an expression of widespread ennui with respect to modern consumer culture, the depiction of consumption in the medical students' graphic novels is important to consider. Caffeine is the medical students' equivalent of the zombies' listless compulsion for consuming human flesh. Depictions of coffee consumption are common within the medical students' graphic narratives, often with close attention paid to depicting the branding of the coffee through the placement of corporate logos such as Starbucks. This is seen in Stamatis Zeris's (2010) work, which explicitly presents his interviews for psychiatric residency programs as a horror story (complete with gory, blood-dripping fonts for the title) and includes depictions of his mindless coffee consumption while only half-awake. It also appears in this comic by Christian Squillante (2009), who depicts the daily ritual of rising for clinical rotations at 4:00 a.m., staggering to the hospital Starbucks, and expediently consuming cup after cup of coffee before rounding with the attending physician.

Almonte and Rupani (2010) also deploy the theme of mechanical coffee consumption, with an anonymous, shuffling (and rather zombie-esque) group of people in line for their morning coffee. In another panel they draw cupboards laden with canned and boxed goods (all presented as being quick and convenient rather than wholesome), with breakfast cereal substituting for cooked dinners.

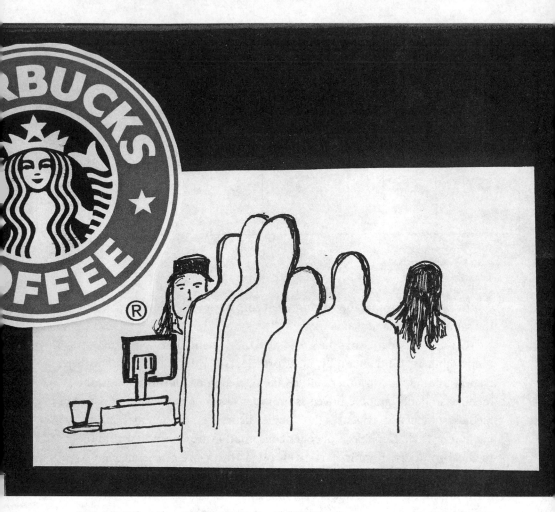

4.4   From Wilson Almonte and Romita Rupa, untitled (2009).

Although the theme of consumption seems to crop up throughout zombie fiction, in the context of the students' graphic narratives, it is less a critique of a wider consumer culture than a reflection of the time pressures inherent in medical education that lead to unhealthy consumption habits (e.g., eating fast food, excessive caffeine intake, and lack of exercise). Ultimately, this seems to reflect the exhaustion and lack of free time for socializing that students experience. Thus consumption is depicted as colorless and devoid of any real satisfaction or pleasure. Eating and drinking, which are (ideally) social events that reinforce bonds with friends and family, become antisocial experiences. Students depict themselves eating and drink-

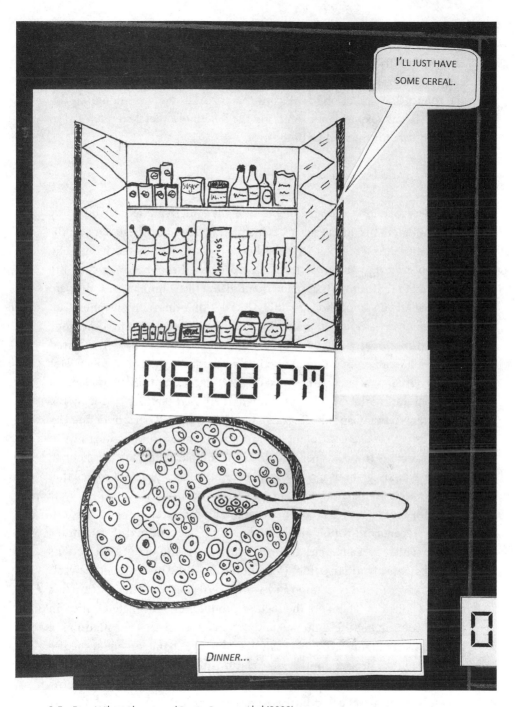

4.5 From Wilson Almonte and Romita Rupa, untitled (2009).

ing alone, in such a way that convenience and speed are prioritized over quality and sociality. Similarly, coffee is not consumed in a pleasurable fashion with friends and conversation but compulsively and individualistically, as a required stimulant needed to simply stay functional. Ultimately, the comics draw attention to the irony that medical students, though studying to become "experts" at promoting the health of others, so often fail to properly care for themselves in the process.

Becoming a Member of the (Bureaucratic) Herd

A subtler trope in the zombie literature is the underlying fear harbored by survivors about becoming a faceless member of a shuffling herd. Once individuals are "infected," whether via airborne contagion or by receiving a bite from an existing zombie, it initiates a process through which they are stripped of the qualities that made them distinctively human, and they are absorbed into an amorphous roaming "herd." After this metamorphosis, all that remains is a body animated by a few flickering autonomic nervous system functions, virtually indistinguishable from any other infected body—a human emptied of distinctive human traits. As the scholar Peter Dendle (2012, 7) argues, depictions of slow, staggering hordes of zombies appeared during the Great Depression and enjoyed popularity during the Cold War, Vietnam, and the Reagan administration—all periods defined by struggles with social control, individual self-direction, and conformity. In many ways, this trope has been deployed in zombie fiction to give shape to collective anxiety about larger social, economic, and political forces that impinge on or threaten to stifle the human spirit.

With regard to the larger homogenizing forces at work in modern society, recent anthropological scholarship has examined the complex ways in which bureaucracies control, manipulate, and delimit the actions and behaviors of human beings (Wright 1994). As the preeminent technology of power in the contemporary world, bureaucracies are instruments of social control that ensure the regular production of expected duties, in part by routinizing the thoughts and actions of workers (Heyman 1995). Indeed, use and abuse of power is integral to the management strategies of bureaucratic leaders and their relationships with the persons they attempt to control through established routine, policy, and procedure. Consequently, as reflected in the zombie genre, the experience of being absorbed into a modern bureaucracy can lend itself to fears about conformity, homogenization, and dehumanization, as well as resentment toward authority figures vested with arbitrary institutional power and control over subordinates.

As trainees entering medicine at the bottom rung of a vast and uncaring bureaucracy, students frequently use their graphic narratives to give voice to the depersonalization and anonymity they feel while expressing resentment toward the authority figures who reinforce the dehumanizing structure. A common narrative finds students encountering ill-tempered resident or attending physicians who maraud through the wards, belittling their subordinates while reserving a special degree of contempt for trainees. These tirades are variously sparked by students failing to remember rudimentary details from their didactic training, making clinical misjudgments, or failing to properly execute a technical procedure. In most cases they culminate with the supervisor marveling at just how incompetent the student has proven him- or herself to be. Occasionally the authority figure will issue threats of what might happen in future instances of insubordination. Tellingly, however, in no comic does an author depict an authority figure deigning to use the student's name, an absence that bespeaks the depersonalization that students encounter.

Through comics, students employ creative strategies to characterize the authority-wielding supervisors who command the medical unit, visually depicting them as different types of "monsters," such as devils in white coats, giant landsharks (Whyte 2013), old, demented men (Yacoub 2011), and, in these two examples, cannibalistic horned beasts (Banbury 2013) and demons glowering from behind surgical masks (Tsui 2011). In contrast, the students represent themselves as yielding obsequiously in the presence of these martinet figures. Depictions even go as far as to show students physically shrinking in size on the clinical ward—undergoing literal "belittlement"—as they are subjected to withering invective from an attending physician represented as a towering giant or as Lucifer (Tsui 2011; Pitzer 2010).

Pitzer feels so beaten down by the experience that he composes an "intern survival guide" with instructions on how future trainees could prepare for the maltreatment of a particularly monstrous attending physician named Dr. Priapus, who was infamous for ignoring, demeaning, spitting on, and browbeating his subordinates.[5] With tongue in cheek, he instructs his fellow interns to "pretend not to notice" when the attending transforms into a monster and begins "howling at the moon." In a similar vein, Lee (2010) writes about receiving a death threat from a surgeon during a procedure and expresses nervous humor about its degree of seriousness. Students seem to

4.6 From Trey Banbury, "Perspective" (2013).

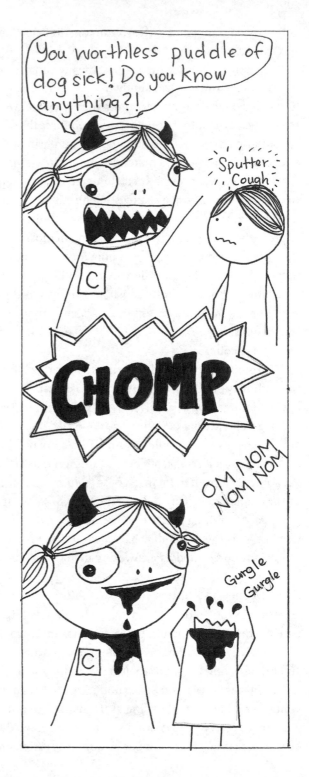

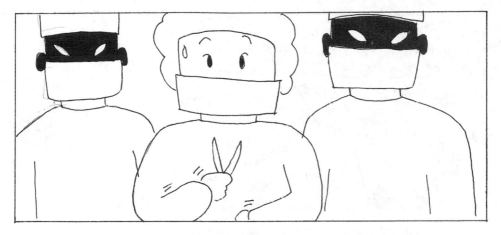

4.7 From Yvonne Tsui, "Adventures in the O.R." (2011).

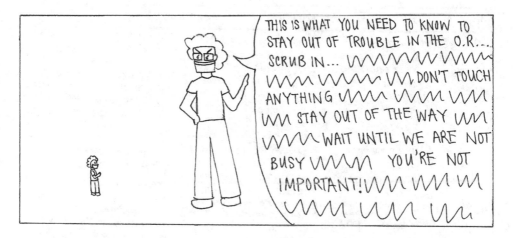

4.8 From Yvonne Tsui, "Adventures in the O.R." (2011).

find particular horror in the behavior of surgeons who preside over operating rooms, depicting these stygian spaces as "dungeons" and dramatizing supervisors as vicious to the point of zombielike violence.

In creating these over-the-top antagonistic characters, students seem to be expressing a deep distress at how their superiors refused to treat them as individuals. The clinical bureaucracy they have entered as medical trainees creates such vast power differentials and "normalizes" such dehumanizing treatment that resident and attending physicians reflexively view students as anonymous members of an endlessly rotating horde of trainees, indistinguishable in every way other than in moments of extreme fecklessness. For

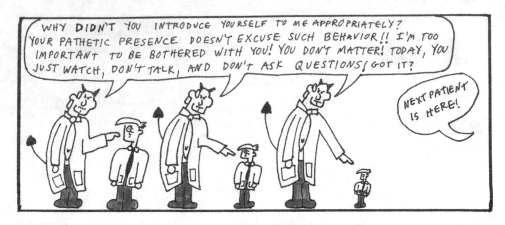

4.9 From Michael Pitzer, "Medical Student: A Tragic Comedy" (2013).

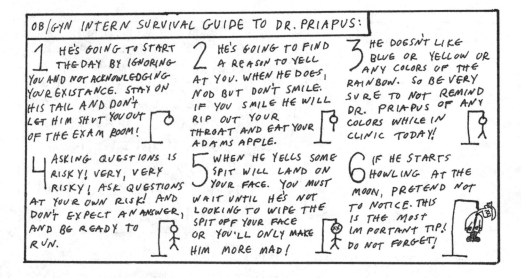

4.10 From Michael Pitzer, "Medical Student: A Tragic Comedy" (2013).

young adults who have always "stood out from the pack" on the basis of their academic, extracurricular, and personal achievements—flourishing within the bureaucracies and meritocracies of higher education—to be subsumed within an amorphous herd due to perceived incompetence and unimportance is a major source of identity anxiety that finds rich expression in the comics.

Even so, some students advance beyond the personal hurt they feel from the mistreatment of their supervisors and examine their attending and/or resident with sympathy. Sometimes, as in the comic by Trey Banbury (2013), this enables them to look past the authority figure's "monstrous" attributes

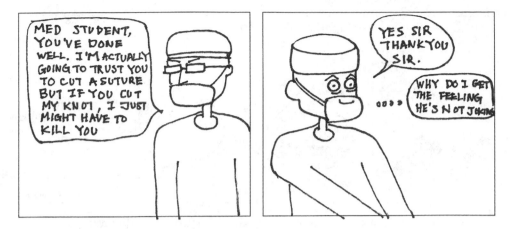

4.11 From Kie Lee, "My First Big Case" (2010).

and perceive them as human beings who are subject to the same dehumanizing bureaucratic forces that impinge on the student.

In creating these narratives, students seem to aim a critique at the wider culture of medicine—a high-pressure work environment that propagates deep disillusionment and antisocial behaviors, not only among trainees but especially among professionals whose lives have long been intertwined with a rigid bureaucratic structure. Students tend to view this institutional culture through a lens of fatalism. Their depictions of an environment where they are subjected to maltreatment by cynical, burned-out supervisors (who have, in essence, become monsters) presents medical school as a mindless machine in which students are mere cogs. These expressions bespeak feelings of helplessness and insignificance in an arbitrary hierarchy, with no ability to push back or call out perceived unfairness and mistreatment.

As in the zombie genre, where survivors undergo a metamorphosis into the living dead, students express self-awareness about the "transformation" of being socialized into a professional bureaucracy that gradually erodes their personhood and causes them to feel alienated from the distinctive individuals they used to be. For students who have previously found education to be a means of empowerment and advancement, the notion that medical school could actively mitigate their senses of professional and personal progress seems especially dispiriting. Moreover, that medical training could produce feelings of such profound powerlessness and depersonalization in students is an ironic contrast to the cultural archetype of doctors as "superheroes" within Western culture.

As I struggled to suppress my pity for her my perception of her changed.

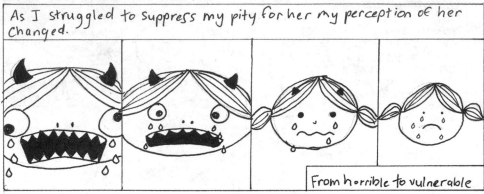

From horrible to vulnerable

Reflecting on this experience I realized that we all carry baggage. Even doctors. We don't always choose what we carry.

Rocky marriage

Fear of aging

Financial troubles

LIFE

Substance abuse

Repressed childhood issues

The important thing is to choose to see each other as we truly are—human beings.

4.12 From Trey Banbury, "Perspective" (2013).

Superficially, medical students do not have much in common with zombies. Medical students are not flesh-eating undead automatons fomenting terror and carnage, and they do not (usually) wander about catatonically. But at their core zombies are beings who have lost their humanity and the essential capacity to empathize. And in this regard medical students fear becoming what the zombie represents—a transformed being that no longer cares for others.

Even more, medical students relate to the survivors of a zombie apocalypse. For both students and survivors, it is important to care about others—but not too much. For it is the case that, to survive in settings of vast human suffering, people must inoculate and distance themselves from other humans in order to function. To truly feel another's pain would be paralyzing, but self-preservation taken to the extreme results in callousness and a loss of human connection. This tension between survival and maintaining one's humanity is a recurrent theme of zombie stories such as *The Walking Dead*, which can be instructive as we seek to understand the range of ways people cope with adversity.

For medical students, the risk of a transformative loss of empathy is particularly horrifying, for loss of empathy is not just unfortunate; it is a negation of what it means to be a doctor (at least ideally). Empathy, as described by Jodi Halpern (2003, 673), is "an experiential way of grasping another's emotional states," and it is critical if doctors are to form effective therapeutic bonds with their patients. Empathy enhances communication and trust, and it influences treatment outcomes. Hence, when medical students find themselves behaving without empathy toward their patients or one another, it can provoke an existential crisis of meaning: can I be a healer if I don't really care?

Loss of empathy is a common concern among medical educators as well (Hegazi and Wilson 2013), and there is evidence that empathy erodes as medical students progress through their training (Newton et al. 2008; Hojat et al. 2009). Thus it is not surprising that students worry about becoming less caring and connected to others and that such apprehensions emerge in their comic depictions of themselves.

For example, in the comic called "Being a Patient Made Me a More Empathic (Future) Doctor," Jason Holmes (2013) describes his own experience of losing empathy during his third year of medical school. As he begins

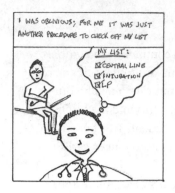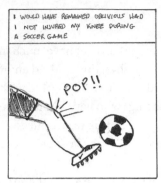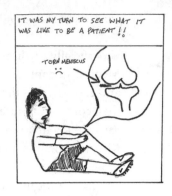

4.13 From Jason Holmes, "Being a Patient Made Me a More Empathic (Future) Doctor" (2013).

to master the lingo of medicine, he starts to feel oblivious to his patients' fears and concerns. In the process, Holmes fails to take the time to adequately explain things to patients, admitting that doing so is "just another procedure to check off my list." Ironically it was not until Holmes himself became a patient following a knee injury that he truly began to appreciate patients' need for information and caring. This particular story has a happy ending in that Holmes eventually learns the value of empathy—but only after experiencing personal misfortune.

Another student, Sarah Farag (2012), similarly reflected this fear of losing empathy in her comic called "The Game of Life." Using the metaphor of a board game, this comic depicts Farag's deliberations as she decides to specialize in obstetrics and gynecology. In the process she describes her impressions of various other specialties that are off-putting, including emergency medicine. When a patient presents to the emergency department with hepatic encephalopathy, Farag asks the attending physician about the patient's prognosis and likely outcomes, and is met with an uncaring response: "Don't know[.] Don't care[.] She is Medicine's patient now!" The emergency department physician is depicted from behind, as a nameless and featureless being that tramples both the student's curiosity *and* her humanity.

Even without overtly referencing zombies, the students' comics often express themes found within zombie literature. The fear of becoming uncaring and losing empathy is particularly relevant to medical students, whose professional identities are deeply informed by a connection to human suffering.

One of the more unsettling attributes of zombies is that they are creatures so depleted of their humanity that the only value they perceive in survivors is the basic caloric utility of their flesh. Zombies are driven by an insatiable lust to consume, seeking out human bodies, violently appropriating blood, tissue, and organs from the living people they overwhelm. Insofar as they have any regard for their victims, zombies view them not as individuals with psychosocially rich lives but as mere ambulatory foodstuffs. To the zombie, living humans are the sum of their organs and nothing more. Recent television and movie depictions often incorporate visceral, up-close shots of vacant-eyed zombies feasting on the bloody corpses of recent victims and lifting still-warm flesh and organs into their clutching jaws. Zombies are a force that commodifies everything associated with the human victims they consume down to their basic organs.

In their comics, students pick up on this theme from zombie fiction, frequently referencing the dark epiphanic moments in their training when they realize their detached "medical gaze" causes them to regard patients as faceless, biologic entities stripped of personhood. However, unlike the zombie's rampantly insensate consumption, the students find such commodification to be quite troubling. This dynamic permeates the story lines in which students assist with procedures in surgical theaters—an experience that places them in the presence of not only an intense attending surgeon but also an anesthetized human body (Lichty 2010).

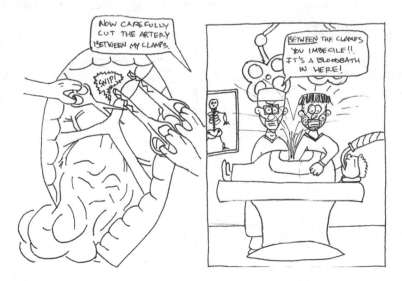

4.14 From Jordan Lichty, "July" (2010).

In particular, the process of harvesting organs from brain-dead patients places students in direct contact with "the living dead" (as one student explicitly references), ipso facto necessitating that they view still-alive human beings as the sum of their salvageable body parts. As trainees, students are expected to actively participate in harvesting procedures, physically interacting with the body on the surgical table by holding forceps, pinching arteries, fetching ice, or carrying out other monotonous technical tasks requiring no (or actively impeded by) emotional attachment.

Narratives often convey the students' initial eagerness to participate in these procedures, but ultimately show the students struggling with the heavy reality of viewing the extraction of vital organs—a living person's heart, liver, kidneys, corneas, and so forth—in terms of pure utility. One student, Nikkole Haines (2011), composed a particularly halting comic titled "A Call to Prayer," detailing this transformation. Upon hearing that an organ harvest of a brain-dead patient had been scheduled on her surgery rotation, she recalls herself thinking, in the first panel, "This is going to be an awesome case with great anatomy exposed!" The next panel shows her in scrubs imagining a cornucopia filled with hearts, livers, and corneas; this explicitly references the zombie genre in its portrayal of one individual's organs as food and nourishment for another.

Her narrative then moves matter-of-factly to the surgical theater, where she watches in awe as the surgeon cuts the patient's body from stem to stern, exposing the entire abdominal cavity, including the patient's softly beating heart, which she touches. She assists in extracting the heart, lungs, and kid-

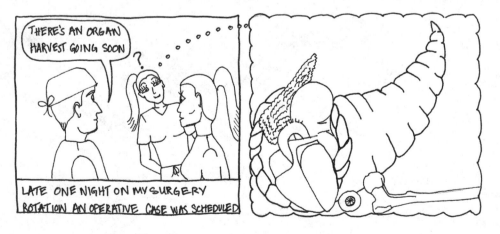

4.15 From Nikkole Haines, "A Call to Prayer" (2011).

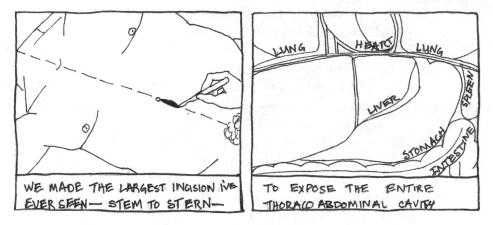

4.16 From Nikkole Haines, "A Call to Prayer" (2011).

neys, which are quickly placed in a cooler and whisked away by a "possessive surgeon," whom she depicts absconding with the organs like Gollum, the covetous character who becomes fixated on an all-powerful ring in J. R. R. Tolkien's fantasy book series *The Lord of the Rings*.

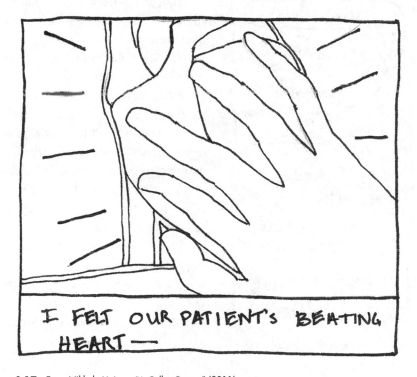

4.17 From Nikkole Haines, "A Call to Prayer" (2011).

Haines initially rationalizes the procedure by tallying the three lives that were saved, but then, as she helps sew up the patient's empty torso, she shows herself being struck on the head with an imaginary mallet as she realizes she has just been involved at the end of the life of a person whose vital organs were just removed. Haines's comic ends with her, slathered in the blood of the organ donor, praying "for [the patient], his family, and the people he saved. My first prayer in eight years."

In addition to evoking anxieties about the zombielike objectifying gaze of medicine, Haines's narrative echoes another subtle theme from zombie fiction where living "survivors" must treat the undead monsters as impersonal threats to be evaded or destroyed. In the zombie genre, sentimental attachment to the undead is regarded as dangerous, often symbolized by cautionary tales about people who are eaten by their loved ones because they refuse to recognize the monsters their loved ones have become. But there are also frequently moments in which survivors, prompted by an unexpected confrontation with the personal effects of those who have turned (e.g., uncovering family photos in abandoned homes, hearing stories about what a person was like), come to see zombies as the people they once were.

In these moments, survivors often feel a hybridized response of guilt and trauma—and it is therefore instructive to compare such moments to the feelings of disquiet experienced during organ harvesting as expressed by Haines. Whereas medical students have, for pragmatic reasons, been socialized into a profession that must treat brain-dead donors as impersonal bodies encasing lifesaving organs, suddenly they have a moment when they must confront the former humanity associated with those bodies. They struggle with quiet desperation to maintain the dignity and humanity

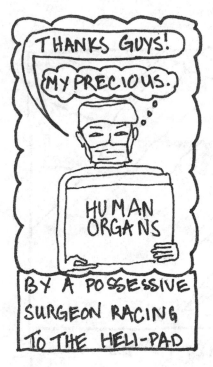

4.18 From Nikkole Haines, "A Call to Prayer" (2011).

of their subjects, while experiencing their medical training as actively degrading their ability to do so.

Conclusion

What do we ultimately learn about the culture of medical school and the concerns and fears of medical students by examining the comics that students produce and the zombie tropes within them? Admittedly there are multiple and interlacing themes expressed in the comics, and most do not explicitly reference zombies or the undead. Indeed, students sometimes choose cathartic narratives that show themselves or their future careers in a positive light. And yet an undercurrent of psychological unrest runs throughout the comics, more subtly evoking, borrowing from, and playing with themes from zombie fiction. In many ways, the implicit nature of these representations makes them even more powerful.

Although numerous zombie-related themes are present in students' comics (e.g., isolation, consumption, emotional fatigue), the overarching concern that emerges is fear of dehumanization. Students express anxiety about the loss of human connection that propelled many of them into medicine in the first place; they fret about losing the capacity to empathize with patients; they worry about feeling isolated and losing their individuality; and they protest being mistreated by superiors within the medical hierarchy. Although students sometimes portray themselves as zombies, more frequently they see themselves as the survivors. While this might at first appear to be reassuring—indicating that medical school is not so horrific after all—it is nevertheless alarming that these students see medical school as something to be survived and endured rather than an opportunity for growth and development. Such concerns are not unique to the comic-producing students; rather, they echo the misgivings raised by medical educators who have long noted the morally erosive effects of medical education (Feudtner, Christakis, and Christakis 1994).

As mentioned at the outset of this chapter, metaphors are "good to think with," and the fact that students' metaphorical thinking sometimes leads them down a zombie wormhole is quite revealing of how the medical school experience shapes (not always for the better) students' self-identities and views of the profession writ large. Ironically, even when given an opportunity to explicitly talk about their concerns and experiences via class discussions,

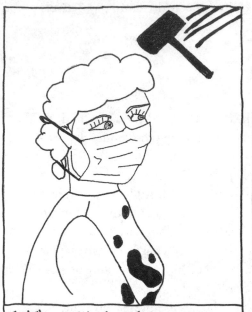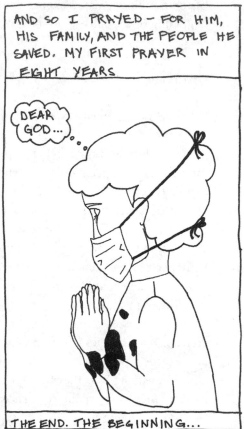

4.19 From Nikkole Haines, "A Call to Prayer" (2011).

these dehumanizing aspects of medical education seldom arise. Instead, students tend to discuss issues such as the patient's experience of illness, how physicians are perceived by others, and strategies for effectively communicating with patients. Tellingly, the darker themes emerge in the students' graphic narratives, which seems to affirm the power of comics to enable people to express themselves metaphorically. As a visually dynamic and disarming medium, comics provide a novel language for expressing complex emotions, conveying simultaneous viewpoints, and portraying the nonliteral lived experience of medical school in ways that prose writing or conversations cannot.

So, what can medical educators do? To read the student comics critically is to understand that their creators are using new forms of description to identify problems requiring our attention. In their panels, captions, and word bubbles, students depict themselves as subjects within an institutional setting that is, at times, dysfunctional, and which—most disturbingly—has the potential to diminish their humanity. As is the case for "postapocalyptic survivors" in the zombie genre, the implicit question inherent in these depictions is this: How does one survive without losing what is most essential to his or her humanity and without becoming a monster? In other words, how does one avoid becoming a white-coat-clad member of the walking dead?

Achieving cultural change in medicine is a complex and variegated challenge, and yet it seems that there is a significant role for medical educators to play in helping students remain resilient to the dehumanization and disillusionment inherent in the bureaucracy of medicine. As evidenced by the success of the "Comics and Medicine" course itself, there is much to be gained in simply providing students with opportunities for creative self-expression in the midst of training that is so heavily science-based and nested in the hierarchical structure of clinical medicine. Educators can advocate for a greater representation of arts- and humanities-based classes and electives in the didactic and clinical years. These educational experiences are aimed not merely at having students engage in the absorption of information (the rote memorization and technical training so common in medical school) but also in the creation experience (activities that are introspective and expressive) using methods that integrate music, visual art, storytelling, and other artistic modalities. These sorts of generative pursuits can help counteract the dehumanizing, depersonalizing tendencies of medical training and give voice to students' anxieties and fears. They can also reinforce professional role development and provide windows of insight for medical educators, as has been the case in our endeavor. Most important, these opportunities provide students with new ways to understand and communicate their experiences using a critical lens, and they empower students to make sense of a professional culture that has shaped students and will continue to do so in their careers.

An important problem identified in the comics is the tendency of burned-out supervising physicians and residents to degrade and abuse students. Indeed, an alarmingly high percentage of recent graduates report mistreatment during the clinical years (Cook et al. 2014). Put bluntly, if substantive inroads are to be made in reforming medical education, the broader culture within which such behaviors are tolerated, reinforced, and perpetuated must also be addressed. Though there is little new about alienation, dehumanization, and student mistreatment in medical education, the student comics shed new light on the lived experiences of those immersed in the medical school culture. And, as with most postapocalyptic zombie narratives, there is no simple cure for many of these problems. What does seem clear is that by banding together to face the immense systemic challenges, educators and students alike can create a more humane medical education model that no longer demands the invocation of zombies as a primary descriptive metaphor.

NOTES

1. For example, see Cottrell (1999); Dennett (1995); Frankish (2007); Kirk and Squires (1974); Kirk (2005); Harnad (1994); and Marcus (2004).
2. For example, see Comaroff and Comaroff (2002); Harper (2002); McNally (2011); Niehaus (2005).
3. See also Gerry Canavan's chapter in this volume.
4. Thanks to Kimberly Myers, PhD, for these prompts.
5. According to Greek legend, Priapus was cursed by Hera with impotence, ugliness, and foul-mindedness while he was in Aphrodite's womb. He is historically depicted as having a large, sustained erection. Priapism, a medical emergency, refers to an abnormal, often painful persistent erection of the penis.

REFERENCES

Almonte, Wilson, and Romita Rupani. 2009. Untitled. In "Graphic Storytelling and Medical Narratives," edited by Michael Green. Penn State College of Medicine. http://www2.med.psu.edu/humanities/graphic-narratives/.

Banbury, Trey. 2013. "Perspective." In "Graphic Storytelling and Medical Narratives," edited by Michael Green. Penn State College of Medicine. http://www2.med.psu.edu/humanities/graphic-narratives/.

Behuniak, Susan M. 2011. "The Living Dead? The Construction of People with Alzheimer's Disease as Zombies." Ageing and Society 31 (1): 70–92.

Bishop, Kyle. 2010. "The Idle Proletariat: Dawn of the Dead, Consumer Ideology, and the Loss of Productive Labor." Journal of Popular Culture 43 (2): 234–48.

Comaroff, Jean, and John Comaroff. 2002. "Alien-Nation: Zombies, Immigrants, and Millennial Capitalism." South Atlantic Quarterly 101 (4): 779–805.

Cook, A. F., V. M. Arora, K. A. Rasinski, F. A. Curlin, and J. D. Yoon. 2014. "The Prevalence of Medical Student Mistreatment and Its Association with Burnout." Academic Medicine 89 (5): 749–54.

Cottrell, Allin. 1999. "Sniffing the Camembert: On the Conceivability of Zombies." Journal of Consciousness Studies 6 (1): 4–12.

Dendle, Peter. 2012. The Zombie Movie Encyclopedia, Volume 2: 2000–2010. Jefferson, NC: McFarland.

Dennett, Daniel. 1995. "The Unimagined Preposterousness of Zombies." Journal of Consciousness Studies 2 (4): 322–26.

Drezner, Daniel W. 2011. *Theories of International Politics and Zombies*. Princeton, NJ: Princeton University Press.

Farag, Sara. 2012. "The Game of Life." In "Graphic Storytelling and Medical Narratives," edited by Michael Green. Penn State College of Medicine. http://www2.med.psu.edu/humanities/graphic-narratives/.

Feudtner, C., D. A. Christakis, and N. A. Christakis. 1994. "Do Clinical Clerks Suffer Ethical Erosion? Students' Perceptions of Their Ethical Environment and Personal Development." *Academic Medicine* 69 (8): 670–79.

Frankish, Keith. 2007. "The Anti-zombie Argument." *Philosophical Quarterly* 57 (229): 650–66.

Green, Michael J. 2013. "Teaching with Comics: A Course for Fourth-Year Medical Students." *Journal of Medical Humanities* 34 (4): 471–76.

———. 2015. "Comics and Medicine: A Window into the Process of Professional Identity Formation." *Academic Medicine* 90 (6): 774–79.

Hafferty, F. W. 1998. "Beyond Curriculum Reform: Confronting Medicine's Hidden Curriculum." *Academic Medicine* 73 (4): 403–7.

Haines, Nikkole. 2011. "A Call to Prayer." In "Graphic Storytelling and Medical Narratives," edited by Michael Green. Penn State College of Medicine. http://www2.med.psu.edu/humanities/graphic-narratives/.

Halpern, Jodi. 2003. "What Is Clinical Empathy?" *Journal of General Internal Medicine* 18 (8): 670–74.

Harnad, Stevan. 1994. "Why and How We Are Not Zombies." *Journal of Consciousness Studies* 1 (2): 164–67.

Harper, Stephen. 2002. "Zombies, Malls, and the Consumerism Debate: George Romero's *Dawn of the Dead*." *Americana: The Journal of American Popular Culture (1900–Present)* 1 (2). http://www.americanpopularculture.com/journal/articles/fall_2002/harper.htm.

Hegazi, I., and I. Wilson. 2013. "Maintaining Empathy in Medical School: It Is Possible." *Med Teach* 35 (12): 1002–8.

Heyman, Josiah McC. 1995. "Putting Power in the Anthropology of Bureaucracy: The Immigration and Naturalization Service at the Mexico–United States Border." *Current Anthropology* 36 (2): 261–87.

Hojat, M., M. J. Vergare, K. Maxwell, G. Brainard, S. K. Herrine, G. A. Isenberg, J. Veloski, and J. S. Gonnella. 2009. "The Devil Is in the Third Year: A Longitudinal Study of Erosion of Empathy in Medical School." *Academic Medicine* 84 (9): 1182–91.

Holmes, Jacob. 2013. "Being a Patient Made Me a Better (Future) Doctor." In "Graphic Storytelling and Medical Narratives," edited by Michael Green. Penn State College of Medicine. http://www2.med.psu.edu/humanities/graphic-narratives/.

Kirk, Robert. 2005. *Zombies and Consciousness*. Oxford, UK: Oxford University Press.

Kirk, Robert, and Roger Squires. 1974. "Zombies v. Materialists." *Proceedings of the Aristotelian Society, Supplementary Volumes* 48: 135–63.

Lee, Kie. 2010. "My First Big Case." In "Graphic Storytelling and Medical Narratives," edited by Michael Green. Penn State College of Medicine. http://www2.med.psu.edu/humanities/graphic-narratives/.

Lichty, Jordan. 2010. "July." In "Graphic Storytelling and Medical Narratives," edited by Michael Green. Penn State College of Medicine. http://www2.mcd.psu.edu/humanities/graphic-narratives/.

Marcus, Eric. 2004. "Why Zombies Are Inconceivable." *Australasian Journal of Philosophy* 82 (3): 477–90.

McNally, David. 2011. *Monsters of the Market: Zombies, Vampires, and Global Capitalism*. Boston: Brill.

Newton, B. W., L. Barber, J. Clardy, E. Cleveland, and P. O'Sullivan. 2008. "Is There

Hardening of the Heart during Medical School?" *Academic Medicine* 83 (3): 244–49.

Niehaus, Isak. 2005. "Witches and Zombies of the South African Lowveld: Discourse, Accusations, and Subjective Reality." *Journal of the Royal Anthropological Institute* 11 (2): 191–210.

Pitzer, Michael. 2010. "Medical Student: A Tragic Comedy." In "Graphic Storytelling and Medical Narratives," edited by Michael Green. Penn State College of Medicine. http://www2.med.psu.edu/humanities/graphic-narratives/.

Romero, George A., interview with Arun Rath. 2014. "The Secret behind Romero's Scary Zombies: 'I Made Them the Neighbors.'" *Weekend Edition*, July 20. http://www.vocalook.com/articles/the-secret-behind-romeros-scary-zombies-i-made-them-the-neighbors/.

Silver, Maggie, James Archer, Bob Hobbs, Alissa Eckert, and Mark Conner. 2011. *Preparedness 101: Zombie Pandemic.* Atlanta: CDC / U.S. Department of Health and Human Services.

Squillante, Christian. 2009. Untitled. In "Graphic Storytelling and Medical Narratives," edited by Michael Green. Penn State College of Medicine. http://

www2.med.psu.edu/humanities/graphic-narratives/.

Tsui, Yvonne. 2011. "Adventures in the O.R." In "Graphic Storytelling and Medical Narratives," edited by Michael Green. Penn State College of Medicine. http://www2.med.psu.edu/humanities/graphic-narratives/.

Whyte, Noelle. 2013. "HMC Safari Adventure." In "Graphic Storytelling and Medical Narratives," edited by Michael Green. Penn State College of Medicine. http://www2.med.psu.edu/humanities/graphic-narratives/.

Wright, Susan. 1994. *The Anthropology of Organizations.* London: Routledge.

Yacoub, Emmanuel. 2011. "August 2009: Pediatric Clerkship." In "Graphic Storytelling and Medical Narratives," edited by Michael Green. Penn State College of Medicine. http://www2.med.psu.edu/humanities/graphic-narratives/.

Zeris, Stamatis. 2010. "The Psychiatry Residency Interview Trail." In "Graphic Storytelling and Medical Narratives," edited by Michael Green. Penn State College of Medicine. http://www2.med.psu.edu/humanities/graphic-narratives/.

5.

ZOMBIE TOXINS

Abjection and
Cancer's Chemicals

Juliet McMullin

Cancer Made Me a Shallower Person by Miriam Engelberg (2006) is a critical and witty graphic narrative about her harrowing moments with cancer. The narrative visually documents the frequent misunderstandings with and insensitivities from friends and acquaintances as people see their own mortality in Miriam's struggles. The horror evoked by cancer is particularly illustrated by her comment regarding an acquaintance's reaction to her after her cancer treatment. The acquaintance, upon meeting her, says, "Oh my God, you're still alive!" She notes those were not his exact words but the horror on his face evoked that sentiment. For Engelberg, the acquaintance's reaction spoke volumes. "When suddenly I became THE UNDEAD" she writes above her self-representation as a zombie.

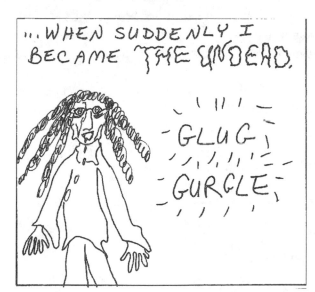

5.1 "The Undead." From *Cancer Made Me a Shallower Person: A Memoir in Comics* by Miriam Engelberg. Copyright © 2006 by Miriam Engelberg. Reprinted by permission of HarperCollins Publishers.

Engelberg's encounter and transformation into a zombie gives us insight into Kristeva's (1982) understanding of abjection and the power of horror. Kristeva argues that the corpse is among the more powerful examples of abjection; it represents the loss of boundaries between life and death, or "death infecting life." Engelberg's representation of the simultaneity of death/life in the acquaintance's reaction to her existence after a metastatic cancer diagnosis can be read as the more familiar fear of one's own mortality (McMullin 2016).

An alternative interpretation exists if we focus on the moment when the zombie is evoked as an abject body. It is not at the moment of cancer's appearance in Engelberg's life, where hope and agency take control, but rather it is after treatment, after chemotherapy. It is the moment when a host of chemicals are infused *into* the body to continue their heritage of warfare *against* the body. Cancer chemotherapies have a long history in warfare. During World War II researchers found that troops exposed to mustard gas had bone marrow and lymph nodes that were notably depleted. This finding prompted researchers to test the therapeutic effects of nitrogen mustard (DeVita and Chu 2008). To this day, Mustargen is used in the treatment and palliative care of certain cancers. The goal of cancer chemotherapy is to kill certain cells so that the whole of the body might live. Consequently the effects of chemical therapy—death infecting life—could be said to be the materialization of a zombie.

This essay is an examination of how the twenty-first century, as a "chemical regime of life" (Murphy 2008), creates and makes meaning of the "ontic/hauntic zombie" (Lauro and Embry 2008). Engaging with an "ontic/hauntic zombie" is Lauro and Embry's thinking around the paradoxical nature of how the zombie is a real thing, an ontic object, and also a haunting ghostly image evoking fear and horror. Referencing moments where language and agency are impaired, historical incidents wherein the mentally ill are treated with embalming fluid, and current debates over life support or medically defined brain-dead individuals, the "real life zombie" is "a material collision of living and dead tissues" (Lauro and Embry 2008, 105) that occupies an ontic space in the world. At the same time, the zombie is hauntic in its imagery, form, and lack of agency. It is a body under the control of another and evokes a haunting fear of oppression and horror. Both the ontic and hauntic form of the zombie, both death infecting life and horror, are forms of abjection. While their reference to the zombie is of a material body, this essay does not consider the individual diagnosed with cancer as a zombie. Rather, I consider how cancer's chemicals are simultaneously the harbingers *and* occupiers of death/life, and thus I refer to them as "zombie toxins."

Zombie toxins manifest at two levels. First, they are unconscious agents that move through our environment and bodies, transforming, killing, and making live. Zombie toxins are haunting in their near invisibility, moving through borders of nation, community, infrastructures, and bodies, infecting and transforming life. Second, zombie toxins, in their transformation of all species, create a materialization of the popular image of zombies. As cancer's chemicals are both life and death, enhancing their embodiment provokes zombie behaviors, an unconsciousness of the body to controlling chemicals that are killing their cells, creating the loss of hair, skin rashes, nausea, and exhaustion that leads to a slowness of movement and mind. I argue that the embodiment of zombie toxins in cancer causes *and* treatments blurs the boundaries of self/Other, of the order that is supposed to be life *then* death, and thus the toxins and the affected body are abject, "death infecting life," or, as Lauro and Embry (2008) would say, "a material collision of living and dead tissues." Further, the representation of the zombie and cancer's chemicals in graphic narratives powerfully visualizes the blurring of boundaries that enhance our ability to see the abject and zombie toxins, the infusion of death into life in ways that words alone cannot.

One of cancer's horrors is that it is not really foreign: it is made out of the body's own cells. However, this sign of death grows "out of control" within your body before you are ever diagnosed. Described as a betrayal of the self (Heurtin-Roberts 2009), cancer's agency evokes fear and a hypervigilant need to detect its presence. Cancer consists of cells that grow differently from normal cells; cancer cells are "mad" and "crazy." Once detected, cancer takes on the status of an invader, not truly belonging to the sufferer. It needs to be cut out, radiated, and/or chemically destroyed. Cancer is abject, and its Otherness, fear, and loss of control must be fought (Sontag 1977). Cancer's evocation of abjection reveals how, as Kristeva (1982, 5) states, the abject is "imaginary uncanniness and real threat, it beckons to us and ends up engulfing us," it is "a terror that disassembles." With cancer, we are made fully aware that we are all mortal. It is in this confrontation with death that cancer patients can be alienated from others and even to themselves, becoming an embodiment of the self as Other. This embodiment is further complicated when we consider the "chemical regimes of living" in the twenty-first century—how "molecular relations extend outside of the organic realm and create interconnections with landscapes, production, and consumption, requiring us to tie the history of technoscience with political economy" (Murphy 2008, 697). Toxins and pollution, along with the chemicals that treat diseases such as cancer, have made us "chemically transformed beings."[1] The tension between the life-giving treatment and the chemicals causing cancer develops into a host of images that evoke both nature (i.e., the normalization of the naturalness of death) and the fact that despite the prognosis you are still alive. Embodying this duality is an example of what Lauro and Embry consider the potential of a posthuman zombie, a state wherein subject and object boundaries are blurred, where life and death are one and the same.

In considering the potential of posthumanism, Lauro and Embry (2008, 87) propose that the "zombie as an ontic/hauntic object reveals much about the crisis of human embodiment, the way power works, and the history of man's subjugation and oppression of its 'Others.'" The materialization of zombie toxins and oppression is evident in both biomedical technologies and the effects of industrial contamination on populations working and living near waste-generating factories and dumping sites. Biomedical treatments for cancer are among the most expensive (see Agency for Healthcare Research and Quality 2012 for costs in the United States) and are highly dependent on technology (e.g., chemotherapy, bone marrow transplants, and the continual search for new drugs). Cutting-edge biotechnologies drive hope for both a cure and prolonged life. But who gets to have that hope when, as of 2015, despite the Affordable Health Care Act, approximately thirty-two million individuals in the United States are uninsured, and high premiums create delays in seeking care? The inability to adequately access healthcare adversely affects every stage of the cancer continuum from delays in diagnosis and opportunities for treatment to survivorship and palliative care (American Cancer Society 2008). Lack of insurance, which is higher among minority populations, is but one effect of subjugating "the Other" through denial of access to the chemicals that prolong life.

Becoming "chemically transformed beings" through the effects of power and subjugation are evident in communities that, because of historical domination, live near and work in industries that generate chemical waste. Singer's (2011) study of a community in Louisiana living near a chemical factory showed a 2.1 times higher risk of developing rectal cancer in individuals who received their water from the Mississippi River versus individuals who received water from other sources, and a 4.5 times higher risk of developing lung cancer if they lived within one mile of the factory. Members of the primarily African American community lived in precarious positions with little opportunity for upward mobility, their lives supported and shortened by their unequal relationship with the factory. This scenario is played out regularly in global interactions, such as the production of oil in Latin America (see Auyero and Swistun 2009 for an example of the oil industry in Argentina), chemical production in India (Fortun 2001), and nuclear disasters such Chernobyl (Petryna 2013). Thus Murphy's concern with the political economy of how we become "chemically transformed beings" is about not only the chemicals that kill us, but the technoscience required to make us live and the unequal distribution of that chemical regime. The causes of and treatment for cancer are a materialization of the "chemically transformed being" molecularly connected to a political economy steeped in warfare and the hope of technoscience. The cancer-causing production and consumption of toxins from cigarettes, household cleaners, and environmental pollution disassemble the body, blurring the boundaries of place, of body, of life and death. By attending to how chemical regimes disassemble bodies and the embodiment of zombie toxins (simultaneously life *and* death), we gain insight into how the war against cancer is organized against the blurring of boundaries of the self/Other dichotomy. Moreover, we can link the subjugation demonstrated by whom we "make live" with biotechnologies and less-polluted environments, and whom we "make die" through increased exposure and limited biotechnologies. I am particularly interested in how graphic novels and comics allow us to see this blurring of subject/object—where the subject becomes cancer's chemicals, the zombie toxins that reveal the imagery that disassembles the body, the object. Finally, since the strength of comics is in the interplay between text and image, I am interested in the role of text in creating a familiar order for abjection and war on cancer metaphors—an order that gives readers a sense of control over the ontic/hauntic nature of zombie toxins.

Following Lauro and Embry's lead, and Haraway's (1991, 152) thinking around the "play of writing and reading the world," comics and graphic narratives of cancer provide a medium to examine both the creation of abjection and the blurring of boundaries (McMullin 2016) created by chemical regimes of living. The artwork in comics simultaneously conveys multiple meanings and expressions of the abject. Kristeva argues that art is a key to investigating the abject. Art allows abjection to be represented symbolically, to expunge the author of the written word's systematizing and ordering of the horror. Text in comics, then, allows the reader to order the images, differentiate between subjects and objects, and make meaning of the world. Language, and the representative text of science, religion, or other meaning systems, give order to the image and reorder blurred boundaries, obscuring the abjection. The corpse is Kristeva's prime example of the abject. The corpse confuses the boundaries between life and our subjective sense of self, and the death of the body (the material object). The corpse is the absence of the self, the ego. The blurring of boundaries and comfortableness with the horror of abjection come about, similar to Lauro and Embry's argument, when we are no longer the agent. Being able to see, to take in the horror and abjection, the "expulsion of the 'I'" that is death, Kristeva argues, can be achieved in art. I argue that the comic, as a medium that plays with the intersections of text and image, is doubly powerful in its ability to represent the abject not only as the materialization of the zombie and as the zombie toxins, but also through our attempts at systematizing their meaning. For example, the war metaphors of cancer's chemicals are a systematizing principle at a molecular level: they help us to make sense, differentiating subject and object. We need chemicals to win the war, to live a comfortable life, to differentiate ourselves from Others. War metaphors are an affect of the abject.[2] Consequently, the zombie toxins become agentive in their mission and the boundaries are not blurred. The illustration provided by comics allows us to see the abject, the horror, repulsions, the experience of being disassembled. Yet the juxtaposition of the image with the text can both put a systematic ordering onto the image or reinforce the disjuncture, the blurring of boundaries in the image (Chute 2010). As a way of knowing and communicating about the world, comics combine text and image such that the interaction creates a "double orientation," a "looking in more than one direction at the same time" (Lewis 2001, qtd. in Sousanis 2015, 64). As such, comics play a unique role in the materialization of the zombie in their simultaneous play of word and image—comics themselves are a blurring or double orientation of self and Other.

Cancer's Chemicals

While never evoking the zombie to visualize death infecting life, Carol Tyler's graphic narrative *Soldier's Heart: The Campaign to Understand My WWII Veteran Father; A Daughter's Memoir* (2015) creates an unconsciousness that embodies the "making live" and "making die" effects of (zombie) toxins. Tyler presents this embodiment in her artwork by illustrating her father's cancer treatment. A series of panels titled "Camp Chemo" describe her father's treatment for stage 2 Dukes' B colon carcinoma. In the midst of sharing the complicated relationship with her father, the pages describing chemotherapy focus on chemicals and toxins encountered in her father's life. The ease with which chemical regimes of life become zombie toxins demonstrates how art allows us to see the abject, the horror, in and around us.

The first panel describing the treatment plan for her father, Chuck, is titled "Camp Chemo Plan, Summer 1995." A colorful illustration of the cabin home in the Adirondacks that Chuck decided to build in the midst of his diagnosis period provides the background for a large blueprint of her father's body. Labeled "The Plan," the blueprint maps out the treatment for cancer and lists areas of his body that have been marred by illness. The side notes pointing to his body include "A. Determined" with a line pointing to his head, "B. Strong & Steady" pointing to his heart, "C. Lungs Clear Despite Years of Cigs, Cigars, and Asbestos." Tyler proceeds to point out where the tumor is located along with the arthritis in his knees. The blueprint of Chuck's body illustrates a mechanical orientation to the body, the body as machine. The body's workings and its emotions can be disassembled into specific parts, with each playing its assigned role. The body as a machine will do what it is made to do. Some body parts can break down; with maintenance of the body, there can be both a slow and fast march to mortality.

The context of the body and the context in which the body is placed illustrates a move between an acknowledgment of the effects of zombie toxins and the figurative creation of walls or space to make meaning of cancer's chemicals. When it comes to the toxins "Cigs, Cigars, and Asbestos," they are recognized as the context of the body, something that is potentially harmful and yet has not provoked cancer in the lungs, which are suspected of being most susceptible to the effect of the listed chemicals. The body as machine imagery and the words that point to the body parts and their roles allows a walling off of the organs. This embodiment of cancer-causing chemicals, or *chemical embodiment* as Murphy (2008) would term this state of being, is particularly intriguing because their effect was suspected in a specific location, and yet the cancer is in a different place in Chuck's body. This does not mean there is no relationship between the toxins and cancer, but rather that the chemicals are thoroughly entangled in the body. The pristine context of the Adirondacks creates a space between the chemicals of industry and the battle taking place in the cells of Chuck's body. The juxtaposition of chemical embodiment and nature blur the boundaries of life and death. If the body evokes abjection, then the environment will soothe that horror by building, naming, organizing, and staging the war against Chuck's cancer. The collaboration of text and a systematic mapping of the

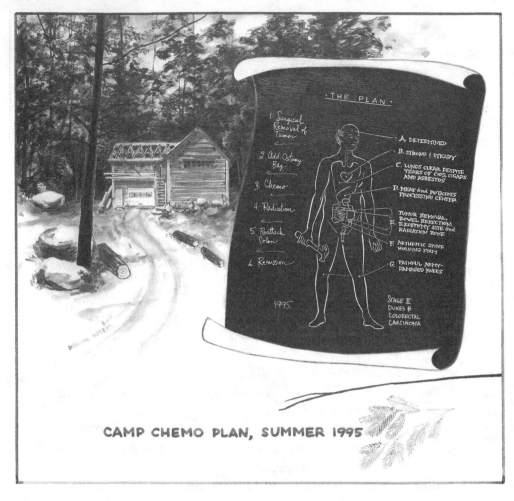

5.2 "Camp Chemo Plan, Summer 1995." From *Soldier's Heart: The Campaign to Understand My WWII Veteran Father: A Daughter's Memoir* by Carol Tyler (2015). Reprinted by permission of Carol Tyler.

body give order and meaning to the visuals of the cabin in the woods and a blueprint of a man that suggest a separation of chemicals and body.

The connection between her father's body and toxins is played out in more detail in two pages titled "The Tale of Mr. Tox-EEK." In another moment of creating a space between external and internal zombie toxins, Tyler describes helping her father move from the old home to the cabin. At the old home, she cleans out a garage full of chemicals used to "clean" the house, the garage itself, and bodies. Illustrated in a brown and yellow-green haze that evokes chemotherapy's military history with mustard gas, the panel "The Morbific Ensemble" shows a pile of rotting canisters, jars, and injection

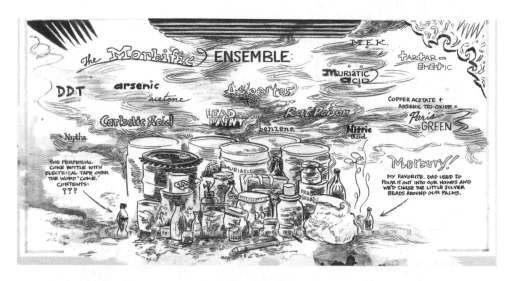

5.3 "Morbific Ensemble." From *Soldier's Heart: The Campaign to Understand My WWII Veteran Father: A Daughter's Memoir* by Carol Tyler (2015). Reprinted by permission of Carol Tyler.

tubes shown with the words "DDT," "arsenic," "Asbestos," "Lead Paint," "Rat Poison," "benzene," "The perpetual coke bottle with electrical tape over the word 'coke' contents: ???" and "Mercury! My favorite. Dad used to pour it out into our hands and we'd chase the little silver beads around our palms." The brown and green haze bleeds out of the borders of the panel, into the gutters, and onto the page. The zombie toxins cannot be contained in their jars and cans, nor on the page; chemical regimes of life form the basis of this set of panels. On the next page of the comic Tyler, tasked with getting rid of the toxins, notes that "any self-respecting 'boy mechanic' type, raised in the 1920s, was bound to have a collection like this amassed over the years." Upon her arrival at the dump she sees the heaps of toxins left for our landfills, the toxic cloud from the can she is carrying trails behind her and again off the panel and into the gutter of the page. In the bottom corner of the landfill we see her father receiving chemotherapy. Carol is standing behind him relaying the story to the nurse. The nurse states, "Oh, I see . . . 'Mister Toxic.' Y'know you coulda just brought that stuff up here! We'd fix you right up!" The toxins here are marked by their incorporation with the body; the cancer cells (not where you would expect them) are destroyed by the chemicals that kill; the borders of death in life are confounded, leaky, and blurred. This scenario is not only a chain of toxic effects but a system of political and economic relations linked to individual bodies. The historical significance of being raised in the 1920s and the need to have a host of chemicals for modern life, that ultimately end up in the landfill, polluting the landscape, making life untenable, and finally as chemicals for Chuck's body as something that would make him live, are intimate parts of becoming chemically transformed beings. This system is disguised so that the transformation of our bodies is unconscious and inevitable. Tyler's representation of cancer's chemicals, the zombie toxins, evokes the abject, where chemicals infect the world around us: transforming life, ending life, giving life. And yet the text systematizes these contradictions, ordering the chemicals and their value and giving us permission to turn away from the horror. The historical and global connections are made natural and unconscious as the uncanniness of the toxins imaged in the artwork elide the subject/object dichotomy, giving way to zombie toxins that make live and make die and allowing us to see the horror.

Agency and Zombie Toxins

Cancer Vixen (2006) is a graphic narrative of Marisa Acocella Marchetto's diagnosis of and treatment for breast cancer. Her book contains more pages of detailed information and illustration about chemotherapy than do most cancer graphic narratives. This detail facilitates a consideration of the internal effects of zombie toxins on the body. As one of the common frontline treatments for cancer, chemotherapy is designed to damage and kill both healthy and cancerous cells so that the cancerous ones stop multiplying. As a basic bodily process, the failure of cells to divide causes a host of problems such as rashes, loss of hair, and pain. Marchetto visualizes many of her concerns about chemo: concerns about not being able to have children, weight gain, "chemo farts," and many other side effects. Ultimately, because it was the best procedure for her cancer, Marchetto's physician decided she would undergo low-dose chemo. This decision was, in part, a relief for Marchetto because now she would not lose her hair, giving her a moment where she could imagine maintaining her vixen identity as the toxins do their work.

Concerns about what her body would do and look like as she received chemotherapy were coupled with contradictory advice from an assortment of medical professionals. For example, her nutritionists told her to eat lots of soy, while her oncologist told her to avoid soy. Also, she should stay away from antioxidants because of their effects on cell division; the goal of chemotherapy is to kill cells, not enhance their replication. Within the realm of professional and popular advice and what cancer meant for how Marchetto saw her ability to control her life and hence her body, cancer's chemicals thwarted any subjective notions of cultivating her vixen ways as zombie toxins took over. Panels showing multiple voices telling her what should be done, how she should eat, simultaneously show the order and chaos of her experience. When contrasted with her previous flashy New York style, the images evoke a disassembling of the self provoked by cancer's chemicals.

The physical exhaustion of chemotherapy is another representation of how cancer's chemicals create zombie behaviors. In an effort to increase white blood cells, patients are given Neulasta shots. Marchetto describes the effect as similar to "being injected by a truckload of wet cement . . . Imagine that truckload . . . hardening . . . in your entire body, immobilizing you with extreme muscle and bone aches." The illustrations show the slowing of a seemingly active body with strong posture and an easy stance into one that is bent over, sluggish, experiencing great difficulty and pain while moving (Marchetto 2006, 164). Similarly, her description of "chemo brain" visualizes the same slowness of mind, with her face drawn as gray mush as she responds to her friend's query about chemo brain: "Another side effect. You feel like your gray matter turns to mush" (165). While the behaviors fit well with zombie tropes of loss of thought and control, I want to focus on the chemical warfare on the body as an alienation of self while the zombie toxins take over your consciousness and create a chemically induced expulsion of the "I."

Chemotherapy works at expelling the "I" and toward creating an unconscious body, one that is subject to the side effects of the toxins that make explicit the simultaneity of life and death in our bodies. The effects of the toxins appear with zombie behaviors in the sluggishness of actions and thought and in their thwarting of an agentive subjectivity. And yet Marchetto resists the unconsciousness, despite her body acting/reacting through the control of the zombie toxins; her vixen agency pushes her body to continue to have a social life, friends, and family. In the ultimate resistance to the unconsciousness of a zombie, Marchetto gives agency to her cancer cells and white blood cells. Evoking war metaphors, calls for cancer cells to move throughout the body, to engage in rampant consumption and reproduction, are regularly sounded as they attempt to evade biotechnology's diagnostics and toxic treatments (Marchetto 2006, 4, 89, 117, 122, 151). White blood cells, drawn as military leaders, call on their troops to fight cancer's invasion. At other times the leaders command the cell troops to rest so that they might be strong for the next impending battle (146, 156). Thus, from the level of cells to that of social relationships, Marchetto creates a self/Other differentiation (a differentiation that, like military metaphors, has been a hallmark of the cancer conversation), that despite physical manifestations of zombie toxins the notion of death in life must be ordered, and unconsciousness must be combated. In Marchetto's illustration of her cancer experience, aggression is the response of her agency. The disease must be fought, and science gives order to the role of cancer's chemicals. Yet, if we were to examine the illustrations without the words, the abject would appear, the nuances of injecting death into life, its horror and its possibilities. The images demonstrate how cancer's chemicals make cells die, while the text makes the body live.

Addiction and Zombie Toxins

Brian Fies's *Mom's Cancer* (2006), an Eisner Award–winning comic, addresses the zombie effects of cancer's chemicals through the socialization of smokers. In a series of panels titled "Just Deserts" (55–56) Fies moves through seeing a teenage girl holding a cigarette and considers it as "A rite of passage." The next panel considers smoking as "A rite of friendship," where he sees two well-dressed women in their early thirties chatting and laughing. He notices that "their cigarettes are the same length, lit at the same time." In the next panels we see Fies wheeling his mother into the cancer clinic. Fies sees "the walking dead": "Old people with oxygen strapped to their wheelchairs sucking down a cigarette before going inside to let steel, chemicals and radiation pierce the dusty meat dangling from their gristled bones. . . . A last rite." In the final panel we see Fies's back as he continues to guide his mother in her wheelchair to radiology. In a thought balloon he states, "The girl, the women, the dead: points on a straight line. Their weak, willful, selfish stupidity disgust me. They deserve whatever they get. *All* of them." From displays of individuality to willfulness, the "points on the line" are mediated by cancer's chemicals. In a chemical regime of life, these panels demonstrate the power of the marketing and consumption of tobacco literally wheeled into the history of radiation and chemotherapy as addiction and need embodied in individuals embraced by death infecting life.

Fies's elegant expression of his frustration, anger, and sadness over his mom's cancer and her smoking that leads them to the radiology ward of the cancer clinic is palpable, particularly with his imagery of "the walking dead." The anger at "their weak, willful, selfish, stupidity" evokes both a sense of agency on the part of the smokers (since they could have stopped smoking)

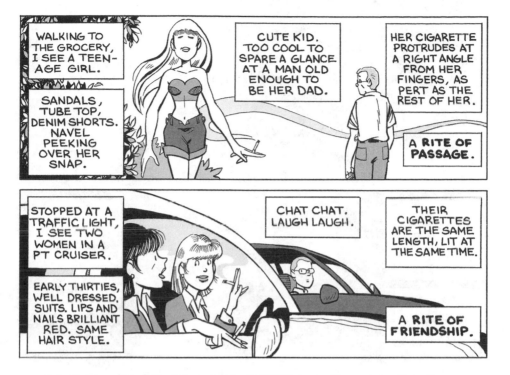

5.4 "Just Deserts." From *Mom's Cancer* by Brian Fies (2006). Reprinted by permission of Brian Fies.

and the inevitability of death from their smoking. As an addictive capitalist hive mentality, smoking and its zombie toxins create points on a straight line. Fies gives us an image of the style of young smokers, from the teenage girl's "navel peeking over" the snap of her shorts and the "pert" cigarette between her fingers, suggesting an individuality and sexuality that moves smoking as a "rite of passage" into adulthood. And yet the daring, risk-taking individualism so cherished by the conscious social being is laid waste by cancer's chemicals. "Rites," while seemingly an individual choice for the smoker, are subjective moments informed by community expectations and institutions. The consideration of zombie tropes, such as the hive mentality, as one of the effects of rites may speak to the effects of capitalism and independence, but it does not allow for the blurring of boundaries that is problematized when the capitalist contradiction is revealed. Much has been written about smoking as a social activity (Poland et al. 2006); thus the contradiction between "willful" and "selfish" is intriguing as a social commentary on subjective representations of independence, which are imaged as the women smoking in a rite of passage and a rite of friendship. Even in the panel "A last rite," the

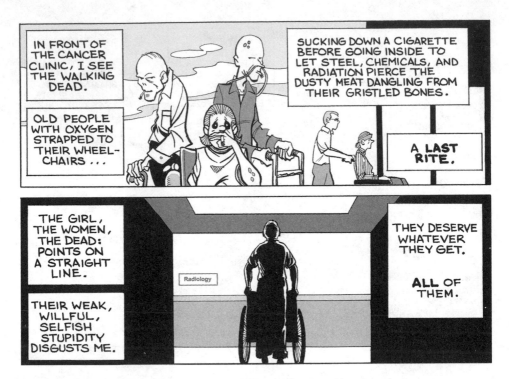

5.5 "Just Deserts." From *Mom's Cancer* by Brian Fies (2006). Reprinted by permission of Brian Fies.

"walking dead" appear to be sinister, highly independent characters. Continuing to smoke signals the need to hang on to their independence and possibly a recognition of their impending death (if they are to die anyway, why not smoke?). Together the "walking dead" breathe in the chemical that has led them to the clinic where, ironically, they will receive more chemicals and radiation that will "pierce the dusty meat dangling from their gristled bones." The materialization of the decaying zombie in people who, once diagnosed with cancer, continue to smoke as ritual is a commanding image. The chronology, "points on a line," suggests an inevitability not just with death but also with the power of the chemicals in cigarettes to infect the sociality of life. Cigarette smoking attracts friends and family to the lack of mindfulness that is usually present in rituals but that chemicals elide. In these panels cancer's chemicals along with sociality come to the fore, and yet the words organize the thought as a multiplicity of individual emotions, desires, and failings. The images acknowledge the social context of our chemically transformed bodies, and the text evokes individual agency constrained by ritualized expectations.

While rites place individuals within institutional life/death contexts, there is also the issue of addiction in cigarette smoking, an unconsciousness of what the chemicals—the tar, arsenic, benzene, cadmium, formaldehyde, polonium, chromium, 1,3-butadiene, polycyclic aromatic hydrocarbons, tobacco-specific nitrosamines, acrolein, nicotine, hydrogen cyanide, carbon monoxide, nitrogen oxides, ammonia, and more—in the cigarettes are doing to the body. Unconscious of their mortality, the cells crave more chemicals. As zombies infused with toxins, they continue to consume, replicate, and transform. Unlike in *Cancer Vixen*, the cells are not given agency in Fies's narrative; only the people who once rejected the public health advice of friends and family have agency that is ultimately hijacked by chemicals. The focus on smoking in these panels demonstrates the power of comics to show the simultaneity of death in life through the conscious act of smoking. The text organizes our reading of the zombie effects of cancer's chemicals in the cigarettes that make the body die and are, in the same moment, juxtaposed with the chemicals in the clinic that make the body live.

Conclusion

What does it mean to create a zombie that evokes the simultaneity of life and death for a disease that has been so mightily resisted? The premise that cancer is a death sentence is a misrepresentation of cancer and death—we will all die, and it is simply a question of how and the mechanisms (economic, political, chemical, genetic) that hasten or slow that moment. The ontic/hauntic zombie in cancer allows us to see how the battle against a cancer death is chemically induced and materializes in zombie imagery and behaviors. The graphic narratives cited in this chapter show us how the chemicals that transform our bodies, challenging our cells to change, are chemicals of sociality *and* individuality. Furthermore, each of the graphic narratives discussed provide imagery for chemical regimes of life, the global and economic connections of cancer's chemicals to a transformation of life. This imagery allows us to see the production of an unconsciousness that argues for the landfill of chemicals, the cigarette that makes a young woman sophisticated, and that call for aggressive chemicals to conquer the Other cells inside us.

Referring back to Lauro and Embry's argument that the zombie raises questions about our historical treatment and subjugation of the Other, cancer is a manner of death that is permeated with aggression toward the Other.

This aggression is most clearly seen in *Cancer Vixen*, wherein cancer's chemicals are enlisted to kill cells at the cost of the body and the effects of the zombie. The war metaphor prevails. And yet the alternative is clear. It is abject. Graphic narratives that employ the zombie call attention to our practices toward the abject. The embodiment of zombie toxins in both cancer causes and treatments blurs the boundaries of self/Other, of the order that is supposed to be life then death. In our opening image of "The Undead" from Miriam Engelberg, we see the social implications of the toxins that affect the body and respond to it as abject. Fies and Marchetto imagine the sociality of the chemicals and their materialization of the zombie. In Marchetto's instance, the zombie toxins are employed to slow her death. In Fies's imagery, zombie toxins both hasten and slow death. Despite the imagery that recognizes our chemical embodiment, the words evoke the battle against the Other, against cancer. In contrast, Tyler's imagery of the toxins that are so thoroughly entangled in our bodies and environments leave us horrified and disgusted at the sight of the chemical regimes represented in landfills. The moment for abjection and a critique of environmental pollution, however, is elided in the joke to invite the zombie toxins to rejoin Chuck's body so that he might live. The aggression toward the abject Other pervades cancer discourse, and it is no different for cancer graphic narratives. This analysis of the relationship between cancer's chemicals and zombies encourages us to change our orientation and ask, What are we battling? Chemicals that cause cancer? Chemicals that treat cancer? Individualism? Globalization and chemical embodiment? Inequality?

The representation of the zombie and cancer's chemicals in comics and graphic narratives powerfully visualizes the blurring of boundaries that enhances our ability to see the abject, the infusion of death into life, in ways that words alone cannot. By focusing on the chemicals in the images of graphic narratives rather than the body of the cancer patient, we can step away from the stigma and the abjection of bodies that force us to see life/death. Instead, we can focus on the connections, the entanglements, the contradictions, and the possibilities. The art in collaboration with text assist us in deciphering the systematic ordering of our life/death through social meanings and structures that work to maintain boundaries created in the horror of a cancer death. This deciphering allows us to ask questions about our chemical embodiment. Ultimately, the juxtaposition of image and text is itself abject as the medium of comics engages us in seeing the possibilities of recognizing our perpetual state of relations with zombie toxins.

NOTES

1. The acknowledgment that chemicals are already present in all our bodies is similar to research on cancer where many individuals understand cancer as already being in every human—it is just a matter of when it will manifest. As a disease of aging, the longer we will live the more probable it is that we will be diagnosed with cancer. Similarly, in the popular Robert Kirkman comic *The Walking Dead* (2003–) the virus that "turns" people into zombies is also found to be already present in all humans.

2. The concept of affect, drawn from Spinoza (1959), often refers to a visceral capacity, beyond emotion and conscious knowing; it is a "vital force" that moves us toward engagement in thought or action but can also leave us suspended (Massumi 2002; Seigworth and Gregg 2010). Thus, in our visceral reaction to the abject we categorize the experience with war metaphors attempting to control and negate the suspended animation of death infecting life, the horror of the zombie.

REFERENCES

Agency for Healthcare Research and Quality. 2012. "Total Expenses and Percent Distribution for Selected Conditions by Type of Service: United States, 2012." http://meps.ahrq.gov/.

American Cancer Society. 2008. "Insurance and Cost-Related Barriers to Cancer Care." In *Cancer Facts and Figures 2008 Special Section*. Atlanta: American Cancer Society.

Auyero, Javier, and Débora Swistun. 2009. *Flammable: Environmental Suffering in an Argentine Shantytown*. Oxford, UK: Oxford University Press.

Chute, Hillary. 2010. *Graphic Women: Life Narrative and Contemporary Comics*. New York: Columbia University Press.

DeVita, Vincent T., Jr., and Edward Chu. 2008. "A History of Cancer Chemotherapy." *Cancer Research* 68 (21): 8643–52.

Engelberg, Miriam. 2006. *Cancer Made Me a Shallower Person: A Memoir in Comics*. New York: HarperCollins.

Fies, Brian. 2006. *Mom's Cancer*. New York: Image.

Fortun, Kim. 2001. *Advocacy after Bhopal, Environmentalism, Disaster, New Global Orders*. Chicago: University of Chicago Press.

Haraway, Donna. 1991. "A Cyborg Manifesto: Science, Technology, and Socialist-Feminism in the Late Twentieth Century." In *Simians, Cyborgs, and Women: The Reinvention of Nature*, 149–82. New York: Routledge.

Heurtin-Roberts, Suzanne. 2009. "Self and Other in Cancer Health Disparities: Negotiating Power and Boundaries in U.S. Society." In *Confronting Cancer: Metaphors, Advocacy, and Anthropology*, edited by Juliet McMullin and Diane Weiner, 187–206. Santa Fe, NM: School for Advanced Research Press.

Kristeva, Julia. 1982. *Powers of Horror. An Essay on Abjection*. Translated by Leon S. Roudiez. New York: Columbia University Press.

Lauro, Sarah Juliet, and Karen Embry. 2008. "A Zombie Manifesto: The Nonhuman Condition in the Era of Advanced Capitalism." *boundary* 2 35 (1): 85–108.

Lewis, David. 2001. *Reading Contemporary Picturebooks: Picturing Text*. London: Routledge/Falmer.

Marchetto, Marisa Acocella. 2006. *Cancer Vixen*. New York: Pantheon Books.

Massumi, Brian. 2002. *Parables for the Virtual: Movement, Affect, Sensation*. Durham, NC: Duke University Press.

McMullin, Juliet. 2016. "Cancer and the Comics: Graphic Narratives and Biolegitimate Lives." *Medical Anthropology Quarterly* 30 (2): 149–67.

Murphy, Michelle. 2008. "Chemical Regimes of Living." *Environmental History* 13 (4): 695–703.

Petryna, Adriana. 2013. *Life Exposed: Biological Citizens after Chernobyl*. Princeton, NJ: Princeton University Press.

Poland, B., K. Frolich, R. J. Haines, E. Mykhalovskiy, M. Rock, and R. Sparks. 2006. "The Social Context of Smoking: The Next Frontier in Tobacco Control." *Tobacco Control* 15 (1): 59–63.

Seigworth, Gregory J., and Melissa Gregg. 2010. "An Inventory of Shimmers." In *The Affect Theory Reader*, edited by Melissa Gregg and Gregory J. Seigworth, 1–29. Durham, NC: Duke University Press.

Singer, Merrill. 2011. "Down Cancer Alley: The Lived Experience of Health and Environmental Suffering in Louisiana's Chemical Corridor." *Medical Anthropology Quarterly* 25 (2): 141–63.

Sontag, Susan. 1977. *Illness as Metaphor*. New York: Farrar, Straus & Giroux.

Sousanis, Nick. 2015. *Unflattening*. Cambridge, MA: Harvard University Press.

Spinoza, Benedictus de. 1959. *Ethics: On the Correction of Understanding*. Translated by Andrew Boyle. London: Everyman's Library.

Tyler, Carol. 2015. *Soldier's Heart: The Campaign to Understand My WWII Veteran Father: A Daughter's Memoir*. Seattle: Fantagraphics Books.

6.

ADMINISTERING THE CRISIS

Zombies and Public Health in the *28 Days Later* Comic Series

Sherryl Vint

By now it is well understood that zombies have become ubiquitous in popular culture, appearing not only in horror and action genres but also as figures of romance (Isaac Marion's *Warm Bodies*, 2012) and its film adaptation (Jonathan Levine 2013), as meditations on the vicissitudes of a post-9/11 culture that consumes its own citizens (Colson Whitehead's *Zone One*), as existential reflections on the meaning of life and nature of humanity (Bennett Sims's *A Questionable Shape*), and as reinterpretations of other popular genres such as the Western (the film *Undead or Alive*), the police procedural (Joe McKinney's *Dead City*), or the comedy (the film *Shaun of the Dead*). In the world of mainstream comics, Marvel created an entire meta-series that reinvented its pantheon of superheroes as zombie versions of themselves, the first sequence of which was written by Robert Kirkman, whose ongoing comic *The Walking Dead* (2003–) was adapted into the highly successful AMC television series (2010–) that brought zombies to the center of popular culture. Meanwhile, the DC Comics Vertigo imprint published the droll urban fantasy *iZombie* (2010–12) series, featuring a sympathetic female zombie lead, also recently adapted to television for the popular youth network The CW. Zombies, of course, have always been metaphors for aspects of the human condition—our mindless consumerism, our lifeboat ethics, our capacity for violence and selfishness, our predatory economics, our waning affect.

Few would contest that zombies have become a crucial icon signifying much about twenty-first-century experience, and the prevalence with which zombies are now understood as a kind of viral infection means that their connection to questions of public health and medicine is also easy to grasp. Among the contemporary vicissitudes for which zombies serve as symbols is the risk of global pandemic, such as was threatened by the recent "avian" and "pig" influenza crises, and this connection is especially visible with the return of the Ebola virus to public prominence given that its symptoms reduce bodies to putrid liquefaction not dissimilar to zombies themselves. Zombies are apt images to convey public anxieties about viral outbreaks for a number of reasons: like viruses,[1] zombies are liminal biological entities that confound our ideas about the boundary between the living and the dead; zombies take over the bodies of those they attack, spreading through a transfer of bodily fluids and turning the infected organism into a copy of themselves, just like viruses; and zombies produce changes in those they infect that mirror the symptoms of viral infections. Recent zombie narratives have emphasized the connection between attempts to contain and manage the threat of zombie contagion and the efforts to control other kinds of viral outbreaks, particularly the recent television series *Helix* (2014–) and *The Strain* (2014–), the latter based on a book trilogy coauthored by Chuck Hogan and Guillermo del Toro. Both feature CDC personnel as their protagonists and, at least initially, conceptualize the zombies as the outbreak of a disease that must be controlled through medical protocols. Perhaps the most noteworthy example of this conflation of zombies and medicine is the CDC's educational comic *Preparedness 101: Zombie Pandemic* (Silver et al. 2011)[2] that uses a fictional zombie outbreak to educate people about best practices in response to real viral outbreaks.

In this essay I want to consider the public education work that zombie comics can do in a slightly broader frame, looking at this CDC comic and comparing it to the *28 Days Later* comic series (Nelson et al. 2014), written by Michael Alan Nelson and illustrated by Declan Shalvey, Alejandro Aragon, Marek Oleksicki, Leonardo Manco, Ron Salas, and Pablo Peppino, which is set in the period between Danny Boyle's film *28 Days Later* (2003) and Juan Carlos Fresnadillo's sequel, *28 Weeks Later* (2007). It follows the experience of a war correspondent, Clint Harris, who wants to observe and report on the occupation of the UK (infected and overrun with zombies in Boyle's film) by the US military (which is "reconstructing" London and repatriating displaced survivors as Fresnadillo's film opens). My contention is that the *28 Days Later* comic has as much to teach us about public health—

and the inevitable conflation of issues of national security with those of viral containment in our biomedicalized era—as does the CDC's *Preparedness 101* comic. Yet, while the CDC comic focuses on individual choices and works to instill confidence in the state's ability to administer and contain a viral outbreak, the popular comic presents the science of contagion enmeshed in the problems of public ignorance and panic, supply shortfalls and rationing, and chaotic violence and military repression that are as much part of the challenge represented by a viral outbreak as is the virus itself. The *28 Days Later* comic series thus presents an image of viral medicine embedded in the complex and contradictory human situations in which this practice of medicine actually happens. Like other examples of graphic medicine, it opens up a space to think about the challenges of viral contagion beyond the clinical parameters of CDC protocol.

Moreover, this narrative comic book, which draws on the other ways that zombies have signified in popular culture, can shed light on some of the consequences of the CDC's choice to use zombies as a metaphor for public education about contagion protocols. Presumably the CDC sought merely to capitalize on the zombie's popularity, to use the familiarity and appeal of the zombie narrative to encourage readers to take an interest in the preparedness training regarding how to respond to a viral crisis. This zombie narrative, however, is polysemic and continues to convey ideas that emerge from how the zombie image embodies our neoliberal ethos of sorting valuable from expendable life as much as it expresses protocols for epidemiological containment. Part of what I want to explore in this essay, then, is the larger set of ideological implications that attend the choice to use zombies as a figure for viral contagion in such educational materials. This is in part an argument about what the text speaks beyond what the CDC intends to say, thus suggesting the need for cultural studies and medical professionals to be in dialogue, and in part an argument about a kind of experiential truth of pandemic that the popular zombie narrative can embody but which the CDC narrative wishes to disavow.

My title is a play on *Policing the Crisis*, an influential cultural studies book on representation of crime in popular culture, originally published in 1978 (Hall et al. 2013). This work sought to study how the public "makes sense" of the legal system and issues of justice through a civic—including popular—culture that represents issues of law and policing, addressing the rise of the law-and-order society in a contemporary UK moving more and more toward the political right. Focusing in particular on the rise of the term "mugging" to pathologize and create a moral panic about crimes of assault and theft, the introduction notes that collecting statistics about such crimes under the new, pejorative label "mugging" had the effect of creating a cultural climate that was more inclined to endorse harsh sentences. Using the image of the zombie to conceptualize the infectious patient, I suggest, may have a similar kind of impact in terms of shaping how the public thinks about contagion and the dangers posed by the infected. The zombie image legitimates an aggressive response of containment in which individual civil rights of the sick are meaningless in the face of the risk they present to the overall society, a logic we see play out again and again in popular zombie narratives in their rationalizations of the need to selfishly privilege the "good" survivors with whom we are positioned to identify. Indeed, the dehumanization inherent in the zombie image seeks to disavow the moral dilemmas that might otherwise be necessary to thinking through issues of contagion and containment, such as the desirability of martial law or the calculus used to measure efforts at treatment over and against regimes of containment, which might include cordoning off uninfected people and exposing them to higher risks simply to prevent the possibility of the disease spreading further. My argument here, however, is not simply that it is thus a "bad" idea to use the zombie to represent the crisis of pandemic because of the ways it can create such an ethos of dehumanization of the infected. Although this is part of the point I wish to make, the more important observation, I think, is that the cultural associations that come with the zombie metaphor can also enable us to think more holistically about epidemic crisis. The zombie metaphor for contagion forces us to remember that there are social as well as medical consequences of pandemic. This larger context for understanding disease is one of the key ways that this reading of the zombie metaphor speaks to the field of graphic medicine.

As Susan Squier and J. Ryan Marks point out in their "introduction" to a special issue of *Configurations* (Spring 2014) on graphic medicine, graphic narratives can often convey through pictures aspects of the experience of illness and treatment that cannot effectively be conveyed by words alone—particularly in the ways that the visual medium can convey emotional and visceral responses, such as the shock of learning that one has been diagnosed with a disease such as cancer, or the diminishment of self one might feel when treatment protocols seem to erase individuality and transform a person into a bundle of symptoms that is monitored and managed by medical staff. A number of these narratives, they point out, call into question "the epistemological authority of the medical profession" (Squier and Marks 2014, 150) through a structure that highlights the patient's perspective, conveying aspects of the experience of diagnosis and treatment that exceed or are seen as irrelevant to the discourse of official medicine. Many contributors to the issue echo this idea that it is the combination of pictures and words inherent in the graphic form that enables it to speak a truth that supplements official medical discourse. For example, Nancy K. Miller (2014, 211) talks about her motivations for processing her experience of cancer in graphic form, explaining that "not only did words suddenly not seem enough, but I felt a strong aversion to the conventional language surrounding the disease and that would decide my fate." Similarly, in an essay analyzing such cancer narratives, Emily Waples (2014, 158) argues that they demonstrate the relationships among "embodied trauma, narrative, and visuality" that is an often-unacknowledged aspect of the disease.

The tension between the CDC's version of public education via zombies in its comic book and the more violent and visceral version we see in the *28 Days Later* series likewise speaks to more emotional and visceral aspects of viral outbreaks and their consequences for public order. Just as the disease narratives of what Michael Green and Kimberly Myers (2010, 576) call "graphic pathographies" reshape our understanding of cancer and orient it away from the clinical perspective of medical facts such as treatment options and survival rates, so, too, does resituating a contagion narrative in the kinds of zombie stories we typically expect to see in popular culture enable us to think about the public health issues attendant on outbreaks in a new way. We begin to see that in public health and contagion, just as in popular zombie narratives, the real danger is as often other people and their responses to crisis as much as it is the danger of the contagion itself.

The CDC narrative seems framed to deliberately avoid the kinds of continuity between pedagogical and popular forms that I am positing here even as, through its use of the zombie metaphor, it also acknowledges that this continuum exists. This tension is most evident in the ways that zombie imagery is used sparingly within the CDC narrative but used overtly and aggressively on the covers for its two parts. The CDC wants to invoke the popularity of zombies to create interest in its contents, but at the same time wants to insist that the chaos and fear of a zombie text is something completely separate from the likely shape of a real pandemic, a separation between fact and affect that—I would argue—thus tells only part of the story of managing contagion. The first two pages of the CDC comic are about establishing the difference between the horror movie world that can "give me *nightmares*" that is also identified as "stuff [that] would never *really* happen" and the real world of events reported by the news. A couple, Todd and Julie, shift their television feed from a horror movie DVD to a newscast that Todd stays to watch, which reports people hospitalized due to a "strong virus" that produces "slow movement, slurred, speech, and violent tendencies." Looking calm and relaxed, Todd then follows the newscaster's advice to consult the CDC emergency website and from there prints out a list of what he might need for an emergency preparedness kit—precisely the actions this comic book, which ends with an emergency preparedness kit list, encourages its readers to take after they finish reading it.

In symmetrical panels that display calm and static scenes Todd begins to gather needed supplies, joined by the patient family dog. These panels do not have any actions that spread from one panel to the next, and there is a sense of a slow pace and lots of time in the transition across the gutters, similar to the film logic of a cut: Todd is shown in various rooms of the house gathering material, calm in each panel, and the abrupt shift of location suggests that at least several minutes have passed as one moves from one panel to the next. A shift to black backgrounds and white lettering for the caption visually evokes horror conventions as Todd and the dog head into the more dimly lit basement, but by the next panel returns to conventional lettering and maintains this methodical pace. By page 6 he has gathered all needed supplies, and his emergency kit is centered in a cell all its own, showing the importance of the supplies and this calm, preparatory activity, minimizing any sense of menace.

In one of the few appearances of an actual zombie in the narrative, this calm domestic scene is briefly disrupted with arrival of Mrs. Clements, a neighbor, who seems to be coming to retrieve her cat but who shows signs of zombie infection. Yet Todd is easily able to push her out the door and lock it, commenting on her ill health and promising to return her cat tomorrow, before returning to the news that is urging people to stay indoors with their doors locked. Thus, far from signaling an apocalyptic turn of events, Mrs. Clements's infection is experienced by Todd as just a slightly more irritating than the usual encounter with a bothersome neighbor. Todd and Julie settle in to sleep in their living room to monitor the news and are later awoken by a number of infected zombies in the street, who are shown close-up and looking at the reader in a half-page panel that doubles as the part 1 cover image. Although the colors and image are darker here than in the rest of the work, the impression of stasis remains: some zombies face out of the panel, looking at the reader, but as many look off to the side; what's more, they face the front of the image and thus move away from the speech bubble attached to the house, which says, "We better turn on the TV," and clearly positions the house *behind* the zombies and thus not as the object of their interest.

Part 2 of the narrative opens with a full-page spread that shows the Atlanta CDC center, with its name and logo prominently displayed in the bottom third of the page and with no zombies present. The following page panels show medical professionals calmly going about their business in this well-appointed facility, and so the sense of chaos and contingency that informs the aesthetics of most popular zombie narratives remains absent from this one. Emphasizing the connection between zombies and the threat of real pandemic, these researchers identify the virus they have isolated as Z5N1, reminding readers of the H5N1 influenza outbreak that was widely reported in the media as possibly leading to a pandemic. In orderly panels similar to those of part 1, Drs. Greene and Chang discuss the status of the investigation as they walk down brightly lit corridors, peering in on neatly organized labs staffed by productive people, with the containment suits standing out in bright red from a color palette that is otherwise dominated by grays and blues, highlighting for us the success of containment protocols. The careful and reliable practice of science leading to a vaccine is demonstrated over these pages, and the only note of urgency is added by emphasis in the text on "staying indoors and avoiding exposure," exactly the message of the first chapter. This warning is pronounced by their colleague, Dr. Ghosh, as the necessary message to send to the public as they continue the slow process of research. Personnel with military uniforms make a brief appearance in this section, but only as logistical support for the stockpile of needed medical supplies to aid in the distribution of the vaccine when it is ready.

Two pages show a brief bit of excitement when we return to Todd and Julie, who have remained indoors as instructed but are now out of food and proceeding to a safe zone as advised by the radio. They plan carefully for their dash to the car, including taking some emergency supplies with them, and although we have a couple of panels that show the typical aesthetics of zombie comics—Julie cringing in terror as a zombie face presses up to her window; a medium shot of a horde surrounding their car—these pages remain in orderly four-panels-per-page configurations without any action drifting across the gutters. Indeed, just as many panels present their preparation for the frantic drive as show the drive itself, and when they reach the safe zone, a local school, they are quickly returned to an atmosphere of order and efficiency, including one panel devoted to the sign, printed on a red background, that notes, "By order of the Wayne County Health Department:

All persons wishing to enter the safe zone must be screened prior to entry." Screened and settled into their temporary shelter, accompanied by their dog, Todd and Julie turn on their portable radio to hear the good news that a vaccine is already on its way to safe zones. The next morning, just as these trucks arrive, the gathered zombies attack the convoy and break into the school, and we see a half-page panel featuring the sort of violent zombie attack we are familiar with from popular culture, which also doubles as the cover for this second part of the narrative. The following page, however, features nine orderly and evenly distributed panels that show Todd waking from this dream of zombie infestation in his own living room. The entire experience has been a dream, and the comic concludes with Todd and Julie planning to make emergency preparedness kits for any emergencies they might really experience, such as the consequences of the thunderstorm they hear outdoors.

This CDC comic has two pedagogical aims: to communicate information about how the CDC responds to a viral crisis and to emphasize to readers the need to have supplies that enable them to stay in their homes in the case of emergency. The last page of the booklet is a list of emergency preparedness kit supplies, thereby conveying a sense of personal agency to readers who can trust—so the narrative suggests—that following this protocol will ensure their survival in an emergency. Throughout, the narrative and visual style emphasize order, thus reinforcing the value of planning and instilling a sense of confidence that the CDC will be able to contain and control any viral crisis that might arrive.

The zombies themselves feature very little in the narrative, although using the two large panels of typical zombie imagery as covers for the two parts of the comic book speaks to the sense of anxiety that people feel about viral outbreaks and about the risks of public chaos as these fears are acted on in emergencies. Beyond the scenes set at the CDC that show how viruses are modeled and vaccines developed, this comic book engages very little with the idea of zombies as a kind of viral contagion, showing no scenes of an infected person passing this infection along, although the frequent invocations to stay indoors and avoid contact with others reveal that the specter of contagion being exacerbated by panicked human behavior haunts this narrative. We might thus think of the CDC's *Zombie Pandemic* narrative as an example of what Squier and Marks (2014, 150) call "the epistemological authority of the medical profession," a discourse that tries to represent the issue of viral contagion without acknowledging the fear a possible pandemic would create. In contrast, the ways the viral zombie contagion is represented in the *28 Days Later* comic is similar to the counter-discourse of most graphic medicine narratives, a discourse that, Courtney Donovan (2014, 238) suggests, participates in the kind of work done by medical humanities scholars that seeks "to reorient the focus of health and medicine away from the biomedical gaze and instead provide a reading of health and medicine centered on experiences, perspectives, and identities"—that is, on the emotional and at-times irrational responses that humans would most likely have in a pandemic, the sort of behavior that disrupts the orderly discourse put forward by the CDC.

Steven Soderbergh's film *Contagion* (2011) might be understood as a fusion of these two perspectives, showing as it does both the careful work of CDC employees to investigate the virus and help its victims *and also* the chaos that descends as humans respond with fear and lack of forethought to the threat of death from contagion—the riots for food and other supplies; the martial law imposed on the city to force people to remain isolated, using violence if necessary; the xenophobic fear of others and the opportunistic crime that arises in the vacuum of quotidian order; the exploitative manipulation of public fears for profit; and the desperate acts precipitated by these circumstances, such as kidnapping a WHO researcher and attempting to extort early access to the vaccine. Soderbergh's film demonstrates that one cannot so easily separate nightmare from reality, hysterical fear from sober assessment of the situation, and thus presents the full set of challenges we face in a pandemic far more thoroughly than does the *Zombie Pandemic* narrative. Similarly reading the *28 Days Later* series in conjunction with the CDC's work provides a more comprehensive picture of public health and contagion than does simply reading the pedagogical work alone. Since the problems of law and order and public panic contribute to shaping the course of a pandemic, the issues raised in the *28 Days Later* series can be understood as a comment on the challenges of public health administration as they are expressed through the metaphor of zombies.

It is almost inevitable that the *28 Days Later* series would present the opposite vision from that of the CDC work given that it is positioned as taking place in the period between the outbreak of infection in *28 Days Later* and the revelation that attempts to restore normality and "reconstruct" London have failed, as we learn early in the sequel *28 Weeks Later*. Nonetheless, it is instructive to look at the particular ways that the comic series represents this breakdown and what this suggests about its counter-discourse regarding the emotional and subjective experiences of contagious infection that are omitted form the CDC's work. Boyle's film was one of the earliest to posit its zombies specifically as a kind of viral infection and was one of the first texts to launch a renewed interest in zombies, revising many of the established tropes for representing them and revitalizing public culture's engagement with this icon. The story of a few survivors of an outbreak of "rage virus" inadvertently released from a research laboratory by animal rights activists who are attacked by the primates they try to free, *28 Days Later* is really about the violent extremes of a patriarchal military leadership who see it as their mission to reboot British civilization in the wake of this crisis. Fresnadillo's sequel critiques the new American imperialism that has occupied the UK, where the virus was contained, cleared away the remaining zombies, and is now "reconstructing" London and repatriating survivors. Inevitably the outbreak returns and demonstrates both the fragility of their rational control and the resulting chaos as the virus spreads. The two films are deeply engaged with an interrogation of military culture, and the latter especially evokes the problems of the American "liberation" and "reconstruction" of Iraq.

The journalist protagonist of the comic series, Clint Harris, links its depiction of zombies and the risks of outbreak to the framework of biopolitical concerns about which lives are deemed to matter and hence are considered "grievable," to use Judith Butler's language from *Frames of War: When Is Life Grievable?* (2010). In that work, Butler focuses on media depictions of armed conflict and the ways they shape our perceptions of war and the legitimacy of certain kinds of violence over others. Such framing of the value of life in war has its parallel in presentations of viral contagion in what Priscilla Wald calls "outbreak narratives" in her book *Contagious: Cultures, Carriers and the Outbreak Narrative* (2008). She argues that "novels and films [and, I would add, comic books] animate the language, images, and storylines of scientific studies and journalistic portraits of the threat of disease emergence," often serving as sites to work out and work through "the anxieties embedded in the chance remarks and illustrations of the scientific, journalistic, and even less fantastical fictional accounts" (257). These chance remarks, she makes clear in her analysis, often portray certain kinds of people or certain lifestyles as the source of disease emergence, obscuring socioeconomic factors, a tendency Wald links to the Cold War ideology in a number of narratives, particularly the film *Outbreak* (Wolfgang Petersen 1995), in which a village in Zaire can be bombed to contain the spread of the virus, but it approaches the unimaginable to do the same to a town in California.

In her reading of *Outbreak* and other films of viral contagion, Wald asks, "Which dead are invariably exchanged for which living?" (262), revealing a conflation of patterns of global and racialized inequity by which American, generally white lives are deemed to matter more than others, almost inevitably those in the global south and generally those of people of color. Boyle's film *28 Days Later* could be seen as either participating in or—as I would argue—depicting and critiquing these patterns through its depiction of a black soldier, Private Mailer (Marvin Campbell), who is kept chained up by the film's chief human antagonist, Major West (Christopher Eccleston), the leader of a surviving military troop who wants to rebuild civilization in his own image. West is triumphant about the difference between this species, the infected, and his own, human. "He's telling me he'll never bake bread, farm crops, tend livestock," West proclaims as he taunts the starving Mailer who, in typical zombie fashion, mindlessly moans and ineffectively pulls at his chains: "He's telling me he's futureless." The only black soldier among them, Mailer also makes visible the racist structure of exploited labor in places such as Haiti, the source of *zombi* mythology; as Sarah Lauro and Karen Embry (2008, 107) point out, when Mailer is later released and rampages through the compound killing soldiers, his carnage "replay[s]" the Haitian slave rebellion that haunts American and British appropriations of this mythology. Fully on the side of the colonizer, West argues that eventually the infected will starve to death and humans can begin to repopulate the planet. Both Boyle's film and the sequel critique this colonialist imperative.

The comic book series extends this critique of zombies as metaphors for lives-worth-saving versus lives-deemed-expendable to the politics of the war on terror through Clint's background as a war correspondent. And this critique can be extended again to issues of how the politics of medicine are shaped by colonial logics via Wald's critique of how outbreak narratives inform such representations even in scientific studies. Clint is critical of the celebratory "occupation and reconstruction" narrative that, for example, is the sanctioned story of the US occupation of Iraq, and in part 1 (issues 1–4) he tells Selena (the black female survivor from Boyle's film) that he wants to go to London to observe the cleansing and repatriation effort from the ground, to go beyond the official story to "things people don't already know about" that lie behind the story told by the "powers-that-be." He asks Selena to be his guide into infected territory and she eventually and reluctantly agrees, seeming to be motivated by a memory of a lost loved one.[3] As the series unfolds, a bond develops between Selena and Clint based on their shared traumatic pasts. For example, later in this same issue they exchange "war stories" as she warns Clint and his team, "You have no idea what it's like down there. . . . You're not ready for this none of you are," and he responds with an anecdote about being in Darfur and befriending an eleven-year-old boy who was later stoned to death for talking to an American. "There's nothing down there I haven't already seen," Clint asserts confidently in a sequence that conflates human and viral enemies, thus reflecting Wald's contention that outbreak narratives often echo imperialist language and attitudes, evident in Clint's depiction of the violence of "Janjaweed militiamen" as excessively violent and irrational, just like zombies.

In the last three panels on the bottom of this page, as Clint tells his story, each frames his face in greater close-up, emphasizing his emotion, but by the final one the frame is so close that part of his face is cut out, potentially suggesting the dehumanization of witnessing such atrocities (cf. Smith's essay in this volume). Later in this section one of the journalists, Hirsh, is bitten during a struggle with zombies, and Selena moves immediately to kill him, just as she educated Jim (Cillian Murphy) in the film that one must instantly regard the infected as no longer human and kill them before they attack. In a half-page panel, Hirsch kneels on the floor and looks up out of the frame as he says, "I'm infected!" the lettering outlined by red to emphasize the peril attached to this status. His position in the frame places readers in the same position as his comrades, looking down on this pitiable figure who cradles an injured arm and looks up in terror.

Selena must fight off the other journalists as she moves to kill him, and two pages later this action is shown in two panels that emphasize its violence: in one her full body is shown in shadow only as she brings down the machete, with three "THWACK!" illustrations appearing in large lettering across the image; in the next, which spans the page width, her face is show in close-up, half of it obscured by shadow, as a mist of blood—a frequent visual motif in the series—spews across the image, which includes another two large "THWACK!" figures.

Far from the images of order, consensus, and calm process depicted in the CDC comic, this sequence is filled with emotion, violence, and irrationality, its panels frequently suggesting motion in the image and at times marked as if they are splattered with blood. The continued parallels with combat situations are one of the ways that visualizing contagion as embodied in the zombie demands we remember that responding to public health crises requires dealing with irrational human responses as much as it does dealing with clinical and medical protocols. Moreover, Selena's iconic image through most of this comic—armed with a machete, in combat boots, her face (and humanity) covered by a gas mask—evokes conflated histories of warfare and disease control, the ways in which the military and medicine

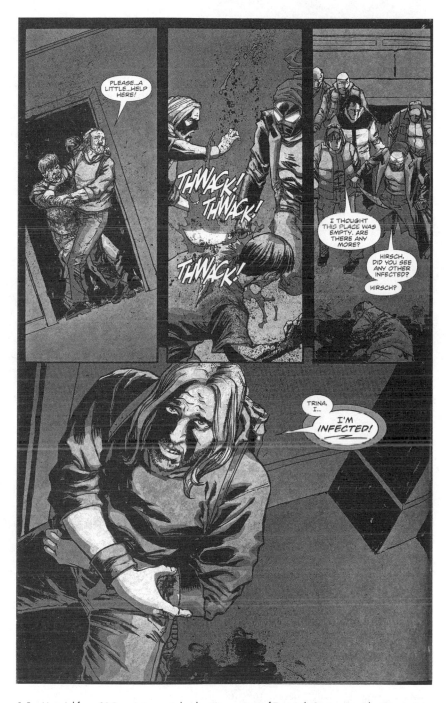

6.1 Material from *28 Days Later* comic book series courtesy of Twentieth Century Fox Film Corporation. All rights reserved.

have been deeply entwined. At times she seems a battlefield warrior, protecting herself from the chemical weapon represented by zombie blood, and reminding us of scenes of soldiers from World War I. At other times she seems like the anonymous and sinister figures in hazmat suits familiar in many popular narratives of contagion who confront—and perhaps dispatch—the infected whose contagion has transformed them from human patient to biomedical threat. The concerns over bioweapons and biological terrorist attacks are always also in the background of this series, and Selena's gas mask reminds us of these connections between medicine and war. It is thus no surprise that near the end of the book, when it seems the threat has been contained and Selena can return to her "civilian" life, she symbolically buries the self this experience has made her, marking the site with her machete, scarf, and this gas mask, creating an effigy that captures the ghostly presence of this alter self.

These parallels with the bioterrorist threat are emphasized all the more strongly in a series of panels in part 2 (issues 5–8), a flashback sequence in which Clint recalls first learning about the situation in London and trying to book a flight to Heathrow to report on it. As they buy their tickets at New York's JFK Airport the panel is dominated by an image of an armed soldier standing at the far right side of the frame. He is not involved in the transaction but is visually larger in the frame than Clint due to his proximity to the front of the scene. A couple of panels later, as Clint continues to wait in line in the background of the image, in the foreground a woman sneezes and the next panels shows that the scene quickly changes to people milling in panic, followed by a panel in which a looming soldier reaches out his hand to confiscate the camera held by Clint's associate Derrick. Order threatens to break down completely in the following panels as the soldier aims his gun at them, struggles with them over the camera, and then shoots into the air to hold back the other people whose agitation threatens to turn them into a mob that will overrun the soldier's position. This scenario—both its disorder and the role of the soldier in hiding information from the public—stands in stark contrast to the frequent scenes of radio or television news broadcasts featured in the CDC comic whose instructions are dutifully followed by Todd and Julie, and thus once again suggests that preparedness for a pandemic requires more than supply stockpiles and safe zone protocols. The entire *28 Days Later* comic series, given Clint's occupation, is predicated on the idea that official sources will hide or distort the truth, and thus its internal narrative mirrors the function of graphic medicine overall to supplement (in the Derridean sense of both augmenting and supplanting) authorized discourses. The recent media coverage of the Ebola outbreak suggests that a comparable level of fear and suspicion exists in the world beyond the comic series as well, and the institution of screenings for fever among passengers traveling from certain locations as a way to allay public fears—even though such screenings were unlikely to identify Ebola carriers in time to prevent contagion—perhaps suggests that skepticism about how information will be communicated to the public is not entirely irrational.

The popular comic is obviously constructing a more fantastical and sinister story line, of course, and is not purporting to be anything like a serious attempt at public pedagogy. My point, however, is that the degree to which such popular images of zombies-as-contagion draw on medical imagery, combined with a general public ignorance about viruses and contagion—evident in things such as the way many people treated the Ebola outbreak in the United States as if it were an airborne pathogen or in a tendency to stigmatize the infected (see, e.g., Westcott 2014)—can result in these popular images shaping and informing public perceptions of the real risks of viral contagion. Later scenes in part 2 of the *28 Days Later* comic echo the clinical CDC scenes about investigating the virus, but here the medical equipment and carefully hazmat-suited researchers are experimenting on enemy noncombatant prisoners (members of the "Crescent Jihad Faction"), suggesting parallels among the dehumanization of those labeled terrorists, the dehumanization of the infected as zombies, and the racialized colonialist history of outbreak narratives, analyzed by Wald (2008, 261) as a "mythic frame . . . through which some landscapes and people are portrayed as dangerous, dirty, and diseased." Like most popular zombie narratives, the *28 Days Later* series is mainly about a number of encounters that Clint and Selena have as they traverse the dangerous landscape to London, incidents in which other humans made desperate by their fear and desire to survive are generally more dangerous than the zombies.

Yet there are moments when the series also reminds us that the zombies serve as an intensified metaphor for the dangers we might face in a real situation of viral outbreak: the dehumanization of the sick who are seen as threats rather than people needing help; the lawlessness that might emerge in contexts of isolated quarantine or massive population die-off, which disrupts local power structures; the uneven distribution of chances of life and death based on class and ethnicity and geographic location. In one sequence in part 4 (issues 13–16), for example, Clint and Selena are talking to a man in Scotland, Raj, who is living under a power-mad dictator who has taken control of Edinburgh and demanded a kind of exaggerated medieval obsequiousness from his subjects. As Clint explains that he is a journalist seeking to cover the story of the repatriation, Raj is almost unable to process this fragment of quotidian normalcy. "Who's the story for?" he asks with bewilderment, and as Clint begins to say, "I've got a syndicated column but there are several magazines that—" Raj responds, aghast, "Magazines? Who's *buying* magazines?" in a speech bubble highlighted with the same red background used in other scenes of intensified emotion, such as Hirsch's pronouncement, "I'm infected!" discussed above. A sympathetic Clint tells Raj that although Britain is quarantined "the rest of the world is *fine*," and Raj seems to find this incongruity almost as horrifying as his experience of living under plague conditions. "Will your story tell the rest of the world that we're *starving*? That we live under the constant *shadow* of violent death?" he demands, and Clint explains that his readers already know these things, but "the world would rather let Britain burn than take a chance on infection *spreading*." It is not that much of an extrapolation to see in this moment a realistic depiction of how contagion circulates in the public imagination by comparing it to, for example, the recently intense interest in Ebola now that cases have appeared in the United States and in Europe, whereas prior deaths from Ebola in Africa had not typically been reported as a crisis.

In part 5 (issues 17–20), Clint's work as a journalist is explicitly offered as a necessary supplement to the "statistics in a cautionary tale of scientific hubris" that he fears will be the official version of the story of the outbreak and repatriation. In a full-page panel, Clint and Selena are shown in shadow only as they stand before a wall of text and images that commemorate the dead and the missing of the outbreak, a wall of mourning that has become a familiar image in popular culture since the impromptu creation of such memorials all over New York in the aftermath of the 9/11 attacks. The stories and images on this wall, Clint argues, remind us that "these people had lives," something that cannot be captured by more official ways of representing the outbreak. These stories and the experience that Clint and Selena have over the course of the entire series suggest ways that zombie contagion comics add to our understanding of the experience of contagion and possible pandemic, showing how these possibilities are experienced through chaotic and heightened emotions, how fear and irrationality are aspects of this medical situation just as much as containment protocols or r-nought rates.

Thus, just as graphic pathographies offer a version of the experience of illness from a patient-centered point of view that often counters the authorized discourse of medical professionals, in the *28 Days Later* comic series we see aspects of the experience of living through an outbreak, traumatic events that are generally not part of the official story of viral contagion and containment. In particular, through its exaggerated tale of military malfeasance, the narrative points to the way it has become almost impossible to disentangle public health from national security issues in a context where the national-security managing of people who are bioterrorist threats is hard to disentangle from the public-health managing of biological threats, as Neil Gerlach, Sheryl Hamilton, Rebecca Sullivan, and Priscilla Walton contend in their book *Becoming Biosubjects* (2011). Indeed, the concluding part 6 (issues 21–24) of the series is about fragility of the return to so-called normality of the repatriation of London, with many of the images showing armed soldiers prominently in the frame. Clint and Selena are no more comfortable in this situation, despite the orderly streets and clean accommodations, than they were in the unpatrolled landscape where they faced continued threats from zombies and desperate humans. One particularly striking half-page panel reports their conversation about this concern only through a speech bubble pointing to their presence off-page, the image itself showing a birds-eye perspective on orderly streets and tiny, indistinct people down below, matching the viewpoint of a sniper pictured in the image's bottom-left corner, his attention and gun, as Selena's speech bubble notes, pointed at "the people *inside* the green zone"—and here we might note that this same language was deployed to mark the territory in Iraq under US military control in that failed example of containing violence and restoring normalcy. Inevitably this order will return to zombie chaos, as we know from the film *28 Weeks Later*.

Popular zombie narratives can thus offer us a way to think about the fear and panic that are part of the real experience of living through an epidemic or fearing that one is about to emerge. The television series adaptation of *The Walking Dead* (Darabont 2010–) comic very explicitly made this conflation in a story arc during season 4 in which the survivors, taking shelter in a prison, were threatened dually by the zombies without and a new "aggressive flu strain," seemingly swine-related, that infected some of those within. Given the story's premise that everyone in the world is already infected with the zombie virus—and thus all will reanimate as zombies when they die, unless their brains are destroyed before this can happen—this story line brought those infected with influenza and those deemed inhuman zombies into very close proximity because the chief risk faced by the survivors was the threat of someone dying in the night from the disease and waking up as a zombie. In a number of scenes during the medical crisis, particularly in the episode "Internment" (November 10, 2013), the shuffling and pale ill people who are struggling to breathe very closely resemble the on-screen appearance of the pale and shuffling zombies. The main narrative outcome of this arc was the choice by one group member, Carol (Melissa McBride), to kill and dispose of the bodies of two sick people without waiting for the disease to take its course. Although seemingly hundreds of zombies are killed without ethical qualm regularly on this show, Carol's choice to anticipate that these two would die of influenced and reanimate as zombies—and thus to kill and burn their still-human bodies before this could happen—is categorized as murder, and she is exiled from the group until midway through season 5.

This narrative arc thus reveals how easy it is to move from a narrative of zombie containment to one of viral containment, from inherently dehumanized zombies to a tendency to dehumanize victims of virulent outbreaks. Indeed, in a widely reported news story (Dearden 2014), migrants from West Africa who came ashore on a Gran Canaria nudist beach provoked a "zombie narrative" response from panicked sunbathers who feared these migrants might be carrying Ebola. Authorities responded by confining the migrants to the beach until testing could be conducted, burning the boat they arrived on, and later transporting them elsewhere in the back of a garbage truck. Although not quite a scene from a zombie narrative, this incident captures the fact that the public response to medical crisis—including that by the authorities—is inevitably shaped by contingency (the controversial choice to use the garbage truck for transport) and fear (the panicked flight from the beach of sunbathers), and that these factors must equally be a part of any outbreak experience. The graphic narrative of the *28 Days Later* series provides a space to show the traumatic experience of living through an outbreak and suggests how much popular culture zombies shape the public imaginary around viral contagion and the threat of a pandemic.

NOTES

1. Viruses take over the "machinery" of the cells they infect to reproduce themselves but they cannot reproduce without colonizing another cell, and so they do not fit simply into our categories of living or dead. Wald (2008, 163) quotes Nobel laureate Wendell M. Stanley on the topic: "Viruses are 'entities neither living nor dead that belonged to the twilight zone between the living and the non-living.'"

2. This document was written by Maggie Silver, with "art direction" by James Archer, penciling and inking by Bob Hobbs, digital color by Alissa Eckert, and lettering and layout by Mark Conner.

3. Although it is beyond the scope of this essay to explore this aspect of the narrative, much of the series is about Selena's transformation from sentimental "girl" to hardened "woman" due to her experi-

ences while struggling to survive the outbreak, and about her desire to return to the "normalcy" of such girl-dom symbolized through her relinquishing of her masculine clothes and machete, emblems of her "survivor" persona, and putting on instead a flowery dress when it seems the outbreak is contained and she can show emotion again. The other main theme of the series is the malice of the military, who are responsible for many deaths due to their desire to weaponize rather than destroy the virus, and whose main representative is a captain who abuses his power in a vendetta to find and kill Selena to avenge the death of Captain West, the similarly insane military commander in Boyle's film who, after she escaped his imprisonment, was killed by the infected Mailer.

REFERENCES

Butler, Judith. 2010. *Frames of War: When Is Life Grievable?* New York: Verso.

Darabont, Frank. 2010–. *The Walking Dead.* Television series. New York: AMC Studios.

Dearden, Lizzie. 2014. "Ebola Crisis: Boat of West African Migrants Sparks Scare on Gran Canaria Nudist Beach." *The Independent*, November 7. http://www .independent.co.uk/news/world/africa/ ebola-crisis-boat-of-west-african -migrants-sparks-scare-on-gran -canaria-nudist-beach-9847973.html.

Donovan, Courtney. 2014. "Representations of Health, Embodiment, and Experience in Graphic Memoir." *Configurations* 22 (2): 237–53.

Gerlach, Neil, Sheryl Hamilton, Rebecca Sullivan, and Priscilla Walton. 2014. *Becoming Biosubjects: Bodies, Systems, Technologies.* Toronto: University of Toronto Press.

Green, Michael J., and Kimberly R. Myers. 2010. "Graphic Medicine: Use of Comics in Medical Education and Patient Care." *BMJ: British Medical Journal (Overseas & Retired Doctors Edition)* 340 (7746): 574 77.

Hall, Stuart, Chas Critcher, Tony Jefferson, John Clarke, and Brian Roberts. 2013. *Policing the Crisis: Mugging, the State, and Law and Order.* 35th anniv. ed. Houndmills, UK: Palgrave Macmillan.

Lauro, Sarah, and Karen Embry. 2008. "A Zombie Manifesto: The Nonhuman Condition in the Era of Advanced Capitalism." *boundary 2* 35 (1): 85–108.

Miller, Nancy K. 2014. "The Trauma of Diagnosis: Picturing Cancer in Graphic Memoir." *Configurations* 22 (2): 207–23.

Nelson, Michael Alan, Declan Shalvey, Alejandro Aragon, Marek Oleksicki, Leonardo Manco, Ron Salas, and Pablo Peppino. 2014. *28 Days Later Omnibus.* Los Angeles: BOOM! Studios.

Silver, Maggie, James Archer, Bob Hobbs, Alissa Eckert, and Mark Conner. 2011. *Preparedness 101: Zombie Pandemic.* Atlanta: CDC / US Department of Health and Human Services.

Squier, Susan, and J. Ryan Marks. 2014. "Introduction." *Configurations* 22 (2): 149–52.

Wald, Priscilla. 2008. *Contagious: Cultures, Carriers, and the Outbreak Narrative.* Durham, NC: Duke University Press.

Waples, Emily. 2014. "Avatars, Illness, and Authority: Embodied Experience in Breast Cancer Autopathographics." *Configurations* 22 (2): 153–81.

Westcott, Lucy. 2014. "U.S. Public Response to Ebola Could Echo Early Days of AIDS Epidemic." *Newsweek*, October 5. http://www.newsweek.com/us-public -response-ebola-could-echo-early-days -aids-epidemic-275249.

PLATE XXI.

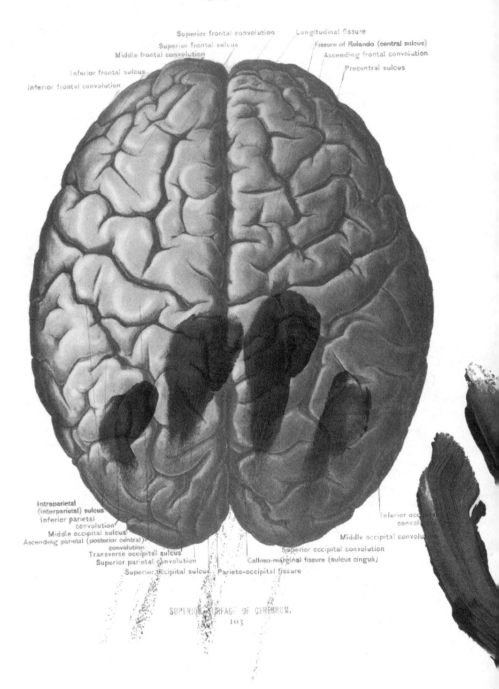

Superior frontal convolution　　Longitudinal fissure
Superior frontal sulcus　　　　Fissure of Rolando (central sulcus)
Middle frontal convolution　　　　Ascending frontal convolution
　　　　　　　　　　　　　　　　　　Precentral sulcus
Inferior frontal sulcus
Inferior frontal convolution

Intraparietal
(interparietal) sulcus
Inferior parietal
convolution
Middle occipital sulcus
Ascending parietal (posterior central)
convolution
Transverse occipital sulcus
Superior parietal convolution
Superior occipital sulcus　　Parieto-occipital fissure

Inferior occipital
convolution
Middle occipital convolution
Superior occipital convolution
Calloso-marginal fissure (sulcus cinguli)

SUPERIOR SURFACE OF CEREBRUM.
103

PART 3: VISUALIZING MEDICAL ZOMBIES

7.

BLURRED LINES AND HUMAN OBJECTS

The Zombie Art of George Pfau

Sarah Juliet Lauro

Corpse Objects

For a long time, I've wanted to write something about corpses. At one point, I even wanted my second book to be about dead bodies, until more than one person (actually, probably closer to a dozen) said to me, "Your first book is on zombies; if your second book is on corpses, everyone's going to think you're a weirdo." Perhaps the topics were too similar: for I was interested specifically in useful corpses, and isn't there something inherently zombie-like about a dead body that serves a purpose? Eventually, I decided my friends were right, and I closed the door on a curio cabinet full of macabre collections of memento mori photography, mourning jewelry, postcards of saints' relics, and catalogs of references to corpses in art, film, and literature. But I remained enthralled by dead bodies because for so long I had never seen one in the flesh.

It says something about the culture and time in which I live that although many people I knew had died, I didn't see a human corpse until I was thirty-one years old. It was the body of my dissertation director, Marc Blanchard, and this was the last of innumerable gifts he gave me. When I walked into the room, I'm not sure now what I thought I would find—only his grieving widow, I presume—but there it was, shaped like my former mentor, tucked in his bed, its eyes fixed on some precise point on the wall, invisible to the rest of us. Silently, I thanked him. But I wasn't thanking him for all the years he'd spent mentoring me, or teaching me how to love teaching and how to "do philosophy," as he used to say. I was thanking him for facilitating this meeting, between my first corpse and me. Death had always been a mystery to me; now, it had a kind and wise face. And I was aware that the corpse of this man, he who had always strove to be only a worker among workers, was still laboring. His body was doing a kind of work for me long after it ceased to exist in that room or in that form.

After that, I started making lists of types of corpses and their uses.

Mostly I was interested in the work that bodies do after they die as medical models or organ donors, as test crash dummies, as forensic teaching tools, as heads on pikes that proclaim victory or defeat, as martyrs or cautionary tales, as religious relics, as political symbols, as objets d'art, as fertilizer. Some of these useful corpses were literally things, as in objects made out of body parts; Nazi lampshades made of human skin, for example, were on my list, along with their representations in art from Sylvia Plath ("Lady Lazarus") to *American Horror Story: Asylum* (the episode titled "Spilt Milk"), or the Tibetan Kangling, a trumpet made out of a human thigh bone, or the calling card case made from the left hand of notorious body snatcher William Burke, of the Burke and Hare anatomical murders that took place in Scotland in 1828. I assembled a kind of Benjaminian Convolute that looked more like the Paris Catacombs than the Paris Arcades, and I called it "corpse objects." On it were things like this poem, "Suicide," by Djuna Barnes ([1915] 1994, 35–36):

> Corpse A
> They brought her in, a shattered small
> Cocoon,
> With a little bruised body like
> A startled moon;
> And all the subtle symphonies of her
> A twilight rune.
>
> Corpse B
> They gave her hurried shoves this way
> And that.
> Her body shock-abbreviated

As a city cat.
She lay out listlessly like some small mug
Of beer gone flat.

Among my collection were corpses that worked by speaking in literature, such as Faulkner's Addie Bundren in *As I Lay Dying*, or that had a kind of power of speech, like the stillborn infant at the end of *The Grapes of Wrath*, sent downstream to tell its story.

But also represented were those in the visual arts, including everything from medieval paintings of Christ's body, to Jacques Louis David's 1793 *La Mort de Marat*, to Gerhard Richter's images of the bodies of the Baader-Meinhof gang, to Richard Carter's contemporary art piece that is a death cast of the AIDS victim Troy Simon Burdine II (1997), to the photographs of the broken face of Khaled Said, the image that launched the Arab Spring. And then I had whole themes mapped out, like corpse tourism, in which I included the exploitation and exhibition of the remains of the "Hottentot Venus" Saartjie Baartman, Sally Mann's body farm images, Andres Serrano's "Morgue" series, and other famous corpses from Jesse James to James Brown, King Tut to the Tollund Man, Jeremy Bentham's taxidermied corpse to the preserved remains of political figures like General Pinochet. And this leaves aside the touring exhibits of real, plasticized dead bodies like Gunther von Hagens's *Body Worlds* and its imitators, and the controversy surrounding the nefarious ways those bodies are obtained.[1]

At bottom was an interest in the work that corpses do and whether that work constitutes a kind of vitality, or "lifeyness" as we used to say in Tim Morton's graduate seminars on object-oriented ontology (OOO) at UC Davis. I found myself using the useful corpse as a way of trying to come to grips with this dense and difficult trend in philosophy. What I took away from those conversations was an interest in thinking about the corpse *as* an object from the perspective of Heidegger's discussion of "das Ding."[2] Because it was lately another object altogether (a human, a being, a subject-object), the dead body was the closest I could come to understanding the abstract principle that all objects have a dual nature, or as Tim Morton has said, "All Objects are Liars."[3]

The object-oriented philosopher looks around the room and every vase, every coffee cup, every chair, every book, every sleeping housecat, every crumpled blouse, every half-eaten cracker manifests the drama between what Graham Harman (2011) calls the Real (withdrawn) Object (the being of the object that we can never access) and the Sensual Object (that we can apprehend). To go into more detail here about Harman's books or about OOO would likely not get us very far: I don't presume that looking at the corpse can teach us about object-oriented ontology even if the kind of mystery that the corpse has—what is this *thing* where our friend should be—was for me a kind of synecdochic grappling hook with which to grasp the difference between the object we can apprehend and that which is always inaccessible. If not the field of vital materialism (including work by Harman, Morton, Levi Bryant, Ian Bogost, Jane Bennett, and others), the predecessor philosophies on which it draws—most notably, for my interests, Heidegger's tool analysis—helped me to better understand the corpse's being, its ontic status and its usefulness.

For the purposes of this chapter, I'm going to focus on one type of useful corpse: the anatomical model. Ultimately, I present the work of George Pfau, an artist who continually plays with the blurred boundary between the living and the dead, between the zombie and the non-zombie, focusing especially on his zombified medical illustrations in order to consider whether all anatomical uses of the corpse suggest that the dead body has an "afterlife." But first, some treatment of the ontological parameters of the discussion is needed.

The Ontology of Corpses

Let's start with a very simple premise: the corpse's "strangeness" results from the fact that it is seen as a broken object. In Philippe Ariès's ([1981] 2013, 586) monumental history charting the evolution of attitudes toward the inevitable end, he writes, "Death has ceased to be accepted as a natural, necessary phenomenon. Death is a failure, a 'business lost.'" In the chapter titled "Death Denied," Ariès addresses the "medicalization" of death, the removal of the community from the death process, and the suppression of rituals of mourning. If death is increasingly seen as a medical failure, the corpse is (at least) the index of that malfunction. But in fact this is true more broadly: the corpse represents our own failure as much as the clinician's, the failure of the body.

Heidegger's (1962, 69) description, from *Being and Time*, suggests the presence of the absence of the broken tool that would later become a cornerstone of object-centered ontologies:

When we come upon something unhandy, our missing it in this way again discovers what is at hand in a certain kind of mere objective presence. When we notice its unhandiness, what is at hand enters the mode of obtrusiveness. The more urgently we need what is missing and the more truly it is encountered in its unhandiness, all the more obtrusive does what is at hand become, such that it seems to lose the character of handiness. . . . It reveals itself as something merely objectively present, which cannot be budged without the missing element. As a deficient mode of taking care of things, the helpless way in which we stand before it discovers the mere objective presence of what is at hand.

The poem I quoted above, in which Djuna Barnes describes a dead body as "some small mug / Of beer gone flat," suggests the usefulness of the corpse for an explanation of this principle. For what object is more starkly visible as "broken," as "a mere objective presence," than a corpse?

Importantly for the syllogism that I'm trying to construct, a broken tool, for Harman (2002, 45–46), is not just that which is "unhandy," but any object that is truly contemplated as an object.[4] However, in a different (and easier to understand) appropriation of Heidegger's idea, Bill Brown (2004, 4) writes of a "chance interruption" of a cut finger, or tripping over a toy, or being struck on the head by a falling nut as "occasions outside the phenomenological attention that nonetheless show you," as Merleau-Ponty says, that "the body is a thing among things." Brown's "Thing Theory" is interested, like Heidegger, in the moment when the object becomes visible as a thing. He writes, "We begin to confront the thingness of objects when they stop working for us: when the drill breaks, when the car stalls, when the windows get filthy, when their flow within the circuits of production and distribution, consumption and exhibition, has been arrested, however momentarily. The story of objects asserting themselves as things, then, is the story of a changed relation to the human subject and thus the story of how the thing really names less an object than a particular subject-object relation" (4). Because of the emphasis that Brown's "Thing Theory" puts on the subject/object relation, it is largely considered incompatible with Harman's *Tool-Being* and work by other thinkers who stress a flat ontology, in which all objects "equally exist"; in this case, the former camp is accused of being interested in objects only insofar as they exist for the human.[5] But my own interest in objects is open to drawing on both approaches in order to understand something like the spectrum of being along which the corpse glides from fetish, as Theodor Adorno might claim, to "actant" in Bruno Latour's terminology, or "quasi-operator" in Deleuze and Guattari's parlance.[6]

Objects normally appear, Brown suggests, like clean windows that we look through in making use of them; we fail to see them *as* objects themselves, until, in this example, the window becomes so filthy that it cannot be seen through properly and the pane of glass itself becomes visible. I want to propose that the human corpse provokes the opposite reaction: it seems as if it is inherently a dirty window, "some small mug / Of beer gone flat," a stopped clock. When we confront a corpse (or even a part of a corpse) it is automatically visible as a broken thing, obvious in its objectness (as opposed to its subjectness). The window of the corpse may become clean and cease to be seen, but this only occurs with overexposure, defamiliarization: for the medical student or the undertaker, the corpse is more transparent than for those of us who see them infrequently in real life. Perhaps for those living in a necroscape like the site of a natural disaster or a war, or a zombie apocalypse, one becomes accustomed to seeing corpses, and they may become the kind of invisible tools that for Heidegger merely clutter the desk blotter.

At first it might seem that the corpse most neatly suggests a reversal of the typical useful object as it is described in Heidegger's Tool Analysis, whereby a thing moves from *Zuhanden* (handy) to *Vorhanden* (unhandy). Whereas the pen, when useful, working handily, becomes visible as an object only when it ceases to function appropriately—when it becomes a useless rod between our fingers, or running low on ink, clumsily gouges into the white flesh of the paper—the corpse is immediately, starkly present as an object (Vorhanden) and disappears only with repeated exposure, as when it is made useful as an anatomical model (Zuhanden). But if the corpse appears inherently as a broken object, this must only be because it resembles a windup doll that has wound down: it has ceased to *be as the object it was*, what we used to call a subject, and it first appears like a broken (subject) object. But it isn't actually that simple: the corpse is a newborn object, special in that it can be visible as an object at the same time that it is working; indeed, its objectness, its new ontology, its perceived brokenness, I'm arguing here, is recognizable as a kind of labor.

Even as it appears as a broken object, the corpse is often put to use: as cautionary tale, as symbol of martyrdom, as relic, as transitional object, a signifier of that which has been irrevocably taken from us; or as mirror, animating our own existential terror. When we do this, Harman might say, we give the corpse a new use and thus obfuscate its original, withdrawn object being. But I'm interested, following Brown, in the way its brokenness *is* its usefulness, for us. We foist onto it a new labor and intent: then, even as it works (for us) it is both working in its capacity as an object, and seemingly not working because it appears broken. I claim, therefore, that there is a whole new category of objects to be considered: Zombie Objects, which work in this manner by means of their affective animation.

As Zombie Objects, corpses are broken objects that are always, in some sense, *working*: to terrify or to assuage, to teach or to warn or to make us remember. True, one might say that they are imbued by this usefulness from the outside, but this is the case with the zombie, be it the product of the witch doctor's wizardry or of a viral plague. By projecting onto a dead body our own fears or uses we animate it with a kind of being: we make the corpse our own personal *Weekend at Bernie's* (Ted Kotcheff 1989). Like a zombie resurrected and put to work in the sugarcane fields, the corpse's new being is not the same as its other being, it is not even the same as the being of the un-useful corpse—if one could imagine such a thing. Is it ever possible to encounter the corpse without making some use of it?

I'll grant that its being is every bit as withdrawn from us as Harman claims of the object and that its usefulness to us gets in the way of our contemplation of the corpse as object. Does an unfamiliar corpse rotting on a hillside strewn with wildflowers have the same kind of being as a medical student's cadaver? Is it the same as the crooked finger bone of a saint? Is it the same as your father, rouged, in a casket? I wonder if it is ever possible to confront the corpse *as an unhandy object*: don't we always find an affective use for its brokenness? Leaving aside the personal element of memento mori photography and a whole host of purposes to which the corpse is put, from traditional medical uses, to curiosities, to artworks that combine the two functions, making use of the corpse in all these matters merely *ascribes* to the dead body a kind of tool use. Some might stress this transmission of affect is not the corpse's real being but just the way we make it handy to us and is therefore not much different from the way we carve the cadaver up for organ donation. But then, what would it look like to imagine that we aren't merely making the dead the repository of our affect, but that some corpses (like that of Khaled Said, or to take a more recent example, Michael Brown) are really capable of speaking to us? If we can think the undead, or the inanimate, as "differently alive," then why can't we apply the same principles to the recently diseased? Perhaps the martyr's body, like the anatomical model, ought to be considered a Zombie Object.

In Jeffrey Jerome Cohen's (2014, 285) meditation on "Grey," he writes of the potential of thinking the undead as "differently alive": "OOO is a nonanthropocentric philosophy in which things possess agency, autonomy, and ultimate mystery. The walking dead offer what might be called a ZOO, zombie-oriented ontology—or, even better, a ZOE (zombie-oriented ecology), which makes evident the objectival status of the body as a heterogeneous concatenation of parts, working in harmonious relation, or exerting their own will, or entropically vanishing, or willfully relating to other forces, other things" (282–83).

Cohen reminds us that "death is a burgeoning of life by other means" (270), in which "the tint our flesh acquires as cells deprived of nutrients become energy for other creatures, for whom our demise is a flourishing" (272). As Jesse Stommel writes in his essay "The Loveliness of Decay: Rotting Flesh, Literary Matter, and Dead Media" (2014, 33), "The human body, even while still alive, is teeming with inhuman cells. Dead bodies call attention to this fact, upsetting the status quo and our sense of ourselves as whole and distinct. Bodies rot, decomposing by means of the tireless work of bugs, bacteria, and fungi. Dead bodies make noxiously present the fact that humans are, at their most basic level, just matter." We must be careful not to confuse the corpse's object being for its undulation with bacteria and other species, its changing over time by the process of decay. Putrefaction is just the corpse's being handy to the worms, after all. Nonetheless, I like to imagine that we can consider the affect or information exchange between the corpse and the still-living human as a kind of "vitality" along the same lines as the body's decomposition into its surroundings. To me, the usefulness of the corpse in this matter is its Zombie Object being.

I share with Cohen, Stommel, and others a profound interest in the way that so many things around us, from rocks and soil to our bodies themselves, are differently alive. In an essay I co-authored with Karen Embry called "A Zombie Manifesto: The Nonhuman Condition in the Era of Advanced Capitalism" (2008, 102) we wrote, "We are all, in some sense, walking corpses, because this is inevitably the state to which we must return," but more than that, we are always already in a constant process of cellular death and regeneration. At the microscopic level, we are always both living and dead, dwelling in "the grey."

The website for the Stanford School of Medicine's Institute for Stem Cell Biology and Regenerative Medicine puts it like this: "Every one of us completely regenerates our own skin every 7 days. A cut heals itself and disappears in a week or two. Every single cell in our skeleton is replaced every 7 years."[7] With the institute's simple sentence structure and emphasis on the regeneration and replacement of tissue, it is apparent that the goal here is not to alienate or terrify those curious about stem cell research; I cannot help but imagine that the authors were trying to counter the sensationalist rhetoric that has so often demonized the scientist as a kind of fetus-sacrificing pagan, wildly dancing around his Bunsen burner. But the specter of death cannot be erased. In its description of the weekly sloughing of our skin, in the vision of the renewed skeleton, in the mysterious *disappearance* of the wound, we are reminded that even as we are continually resurrecting ourselves, we are also, continually, dying.

For me, this passage conjures this image of the flayed cadaver holding in one hand a knife and in the other his own skin: it hangs like cloth, with the face flattened to an abstract pattern. Just behind it lurks this other one, of Bidloo's grinning skeleton holding up what appears to be a shroud. The contemporary artist George Pfau is apparently haunted by these images, too, for he zombifies them and others like them in his work. I will turn to his experiments in artistic zombification in a moment, but first I will consider medical illustrations as Zombie Objects.

William Loechel's (1960) overview of the "History of Medical Illustration" stresses the importance of collaboration in the process, beginning in the Renaissance, in which the physician or anatomist employed a freelance illustrator, thereby combining both medical expertise and artistic capability. Loechel also notes that a great advancement was made in the post-Renaissance development of lithography: "Both artist and physician had begun to realize that not only were their specialties useful in combination . . . but that a third specialty entered into the sphere of activity, that of the printer. All three were striving to get medical education in books of a higher caliber to those who needed them" (170). With advancements in printing technology, they began to see the increased usefulness of their work, its further reach. And yet, to my mind, it seems that Loechel is ignoring the fourth collaborator here, the dead man, the object of medical study lending himself to dissection for a purpose. Whether he has done so willingly or unwillingly is not a factor in proclaiming illustrations of cadavers Zombie Objects, for a zombie has no will of its own, and yet it remains animated beyond its death.

A 2014 piece in *The Guardian* that presents Richard Burnett's book *The Sick Rose: Disease and the Art of Medical Illustration* begins with a quotation from J. G. Ballard's autobiographical novel *The Kindness of Women*, from a discussion of the author's experiences as a Cambridge medical student: "As the four teams began to dissect this unknown woman, opening flaps of skin in her limbs, neck, and abdomen, she *seemed to undress* in a last act of self-

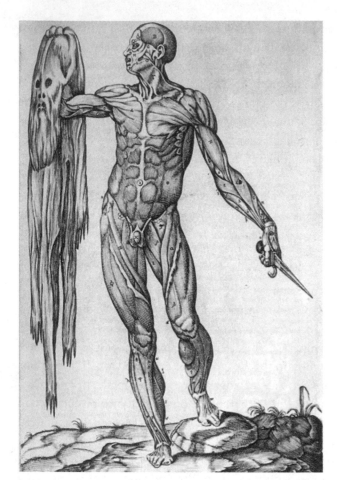

7.1 From Juan Valverde de Amusco, *Anatomia del corpo humano* . . . (Rome, 1559). Copperplate engraving. National Library of Medicine.

revelation, *unpacking herself* of all the mortal elements of her life" (qtd. in Self 2014; emphasis added). Self considers Ballard's imbuing of the cadaver with agency as "disturbing," but this uncanny tension in the depiction of the dissection model is precisely that which we find in the zombie and, more broadly, in the medical illustrator's cadaver: tension between the inanimate imbued with life from the outside and the animate evacuated of its genuine life force that still labors. In his zombification of recognizable forms from the history of medical illustration, George Pfau makes visible this conflict, which exists in the illustration of the dissected corpse especially after printing technology ensured that the images of the dead man's circulatory system would, in continuing to circulate, emulate something like its flow in life.

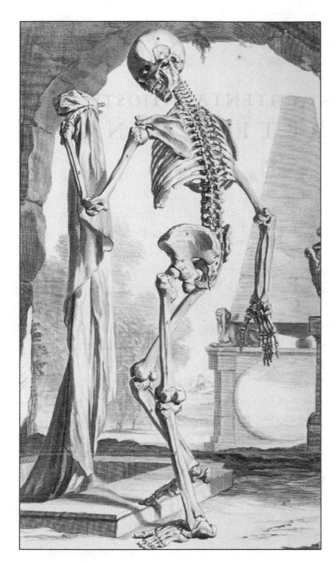

7.2 From Govard Bidloo, *Ontleding des menschelyken lichaams* (Amsterdam, 1690). Copperplate engraving with etching. National Library of Medicine.

George Pfau's "Grey" Zone

The San Francisco–based artist George Pfau may be best known for his "Zombieindex.us" (pronounced "us"), an online, interactive illustration of a pan-zombie horde, containing diverse figurations of the undead from Haiti's real-life zombie Clairvius Narcisse, profiled at length in Wade Davis's *The Serpent and the Rainbow*, to the "hyper-white" zombies (to use Elizabeth

McAlister's [2012] term) of the film adaptation of Richard Matheson's novel *I Am Legend*, starring Will Smith and directed by Francis Lawrence.[8] Providing a veritable panoply of zombies of all shades and forms as well as hyperlinks to a range of websites referencing the zombie, "Zombieindex.us" manifests the swarm, making visible the way our culture has been inundated with images of the undead over the past century and, especially, the most recent decade.

Elsewhere I've written about Pfau's "Zombieindex.us" and his "Zombie-escapes," luscious oil paintings that capture a single frame from a zombie film, rendered in an impressionist, nearly pointillist manner (Lauro 2015). Pfau's intentions here are complex, but the stylistic appropriation emphasizes both the blurriness of zombie identity and the body's breakdown in life as well as death: his use of an impressionist style approximates the diffusion of the body into its environment. He writes, "The landscapes are rendered in oil on linen allowing for a situation in which figures visibly blend into their environment, and vice versa" (Pfau 2013). To emphasize the point, Pfau displays blown-up photographs of the figures in these paintings (what he calls the "zoomed zombiescape" images) in his studio and exhibits of the work alongside the paintings themselves, to show how little each form (human, zombie) differs from its immediate surroundings: a slight change in hue or the sweep of a brushstroke are all that differentiate a human torso from a tree trunk in some cases. Both "Zombieindex.us" and the "Zombie-scapes" inundate the viewer with their color palates and with their uses of depth, shadow, and scale, but Pfau's "Zombie Medical Drawings" series is very different. Consisting of pin-sharp black line letterpress prints, the images seem concrete, flat visuals shallowly carved into the paper. In part, their depth is in their historical referents.

The letterpress prints that comprise Pfau's series of medical illustrations are fifteen-by-eleven-inch "mash-ups" that have points of reference in both pre-x-ray bodily imaging, like Renaissance-era artists such as Andreas Vesalius, and works of contemporary fiction (Pfau 2014). Though each one of the prints is starkly different from the next, what they have in common is an emphasis on the thin black line of the image's construction. I'll go through this series quickly, as if laying out some terrible tarot reading. As we proceed through the images, in an order I have assigned, we will see how they become distanced from the model of the anatomical illustration in a way similar to Pfau's other experiments in abstraction with the human form.

In the piece titled "iI (Organ Removal)" (fig. 7.3) from this series we see the images above (figs. 7.1 and 7.2) called forth again before our eyes. The

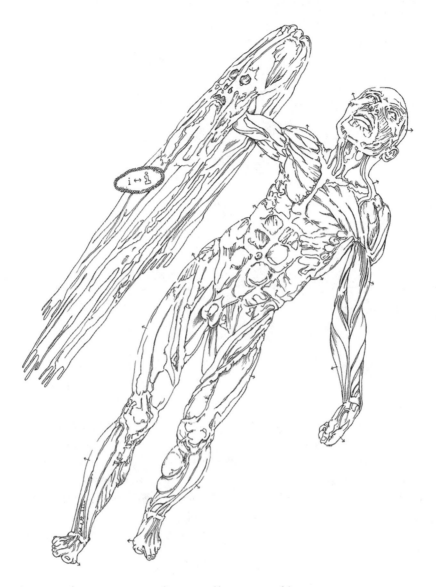

7.3 George Pfau, "il (Organ Removal)." Reprinted by permission of the artist.

piece directly refers to the zombie protagonist Big Daddy from the 2005 George Romero film *Land of the Dead* (Pfau 2014). It also obviously and explicitly references the trope of the man holding his own skin, as in Gaspar Becerra's 1556 etching (fig. 7.1), repeated in Damien Hirst's contemporary sculpture of Saint Bartholomew as well as predecessor depictions of the flayed martyr, and in Gunther von Hagens's currently touring *Body Worlds* exhibit. The images of the man holding his own skin have always reminded

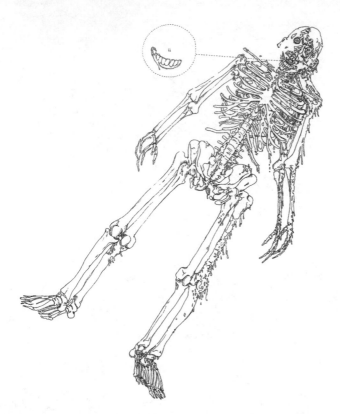

7.4 George Pfau, "ii (Merged Facades)." Reprinted by permission of the artist.

me of the trope of the resurrected corpse holding his shroud, giving a kind of mis-en-abîme effect to the layered references. Of the series, Pfau (2014) writes, "Zombies and the living people that they bite are often cloaked in extra layers of skin or flesh, prosthetic costumes, often placing 'outside and inside' on top of another 'outside and inside.'" A similar theme is lined out in the print titled "ii (Merged Facades)" (fig. 7.4).

This image is based on the "Tarman" zombie from Dan O'Bannon's 1985 film *The Return of the Living Dead*. It is rendered as a skeletal study of a figure that, in the film, is primordially oozing, dripping flesh that hangs in ribbons. But the illustration here is also itself uncannily doubled, like a mistake in film development. A circular inset provides a close-up of the teeth, labeled "ii." Pfau has said that the inspiration for the work was an error in the film's construction—in one pivotal scene, the actor's teeth can be seen behind the false teeth of the costume. Tarman's excessive materiality thus extends beyond the frame of the fictional narrative, as a grotesque set of remains preserved in ooze, to the double embodiment of the costumed actor. Because Pfau is, at every turn, concerned with the blurred boundary lines between the body and the space around it, between delineations of self and

7.5 George Pfau, "Zombie, Examined." Reprinted by permission of the artist.

Other, and between life and death, these visual meditations reflect on the parity between the zombie's overtly messy embodiment and the human's innately blurred borders. In this series, he takes aim specifically at medical illustrations as zombielike objects, for the way they preserve the life of the initial dissection subject and, often, depict that subject as animate, offering itself to the viewer.

"Zombie, Examined" (fig. 7.5) takes the head of zombie Number 9 (the cheerleader) from *Land of the Dead* for this study of the vascular system, which borrows directly from Charles Estienne's 1546 woodcut, *La dissection des parties du corps humain* (fig. 7.6). But whereas the skeletal model in the original holds the lower pan of his jaw in his right hand (at first I thought it was a little boat), Pfau's zombification holds her own brain. As in the original, index lines sprout from the body, marking sections with lowercase roman numerals, as if there is meant to be an accompanying key, gesturing to where, in a textbook, one might find Latin names: "v. cava superior," "a carotis communis," "v. femoralis." But if this image is a cross-section of a zombie and Estienne's anatomical woodcut, it also recalls a portrait of a saint: the removal of the brain and the heart, situated alongside her body, remind me

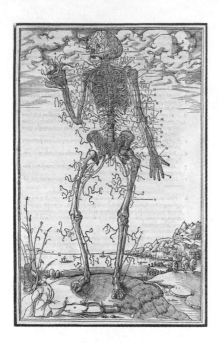

7.6 From Charles Estienne and Étienne de la Rivière, *La dissection des parties du corps humain* (Paris, 1546). Woodcut. National Library of Medicine.

of the postures of some Christian martyrs, like Saint Lucy, who is often depicted holding her own eyeballs. The figure gazes heavenward, holding her brain by its stem, and gestures to an enlarged heart shown from four points of view; it even looks as if she is wearing some type of veil, though the body is naked, stripped of her skin and flesh. It may be portraying the medical subject as sacrifice, which we see even in the postures of the originals, like the man holding his own skin and its allusion to the flayed St. Bartholomew.

"Penetrated Core (Continued Functioning?)" borrows its zombie from Romero's 1978 *Dawn of the Dead* (Pfau 2014). Here Pfau draws again on another classical anatomical posture, of the man or woman peeling back his or her skin to reveal innards, womb, or musculature for the viewer's gaze, as in John Browne's 1681 *A Complete treatise of the muscles* or, more directly, Guilio Casserio's 1627 copperplate engraving *Tabulae Anatomicae* (fig. 7.8). The copy of the latter figure's posture here is precise, as it holds its flap of skin open in a delicate gesture, with three fingers extended.

This delicacy concretizes a larger point that Pfau's work makes about the aesthetics of the open body,[9] but it also echoes the sentiment underscored in Ballard's description of the dissection: the subject offers itself to the viewer. At one and the same time, there is violence and beauty in these images that conflate the inside and the outside, the object of medical study and the agentic subject. And, as in Pfau's "Zombiescapes," his points of reference cast shadows back on the originals he chooses to zombify. Unlike Pfau's revisions, in which the figures are etched into white space, surrounded only by their own organs and the index lines or numerals that make notations on their bodies, his predecessors depicted their figures within the conventions of landscape portraiture: these grotesque bodies stand, in the original medical

7.7 George Pfau, "Penetrated Core (Continued Functioning?)." Reprinted by permission of the artist.

illustrations, on a hillside or under stormy skies. By removing this context, Pfau's work underlines an important question: What was behind the choice to depict the early anatomical models as still living or animated? Was it merely to underscore the point that all living beings walking around had these hidden parts beneath their skin? Was it to obfuscate the bleak reality of how anatomists were able to complete such studies, by working with cadavers?[10] Or does it suggest that the anatomical model, by means of its use in these artists' study, obtained a kind of life after death?

Other letterpress images created by Pfau may or may not be considered directly a part of the medical illustration series, yet they each play with the human form, identity, and the conventions of illustration. "(Dis)assembled," for example, takes its figure from Romero's *Day of the Dead,* although even the most well-educated zombie film fan would struggle to identify him, for the point here is to emphasize that "identity transforms as recognizable features peel away, [and the] specific becomes generalized and grotesque" (Pfau 2013).

Pfau's interest in the topic—detected not only by spending time with his work as I've done over the past few years, but also by reading his insightful

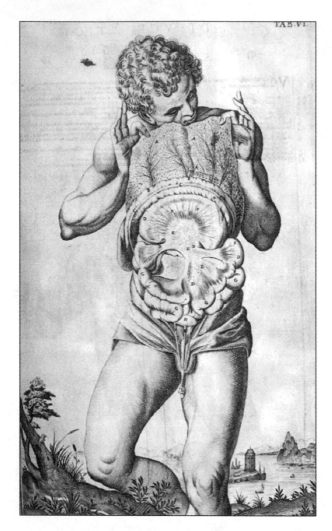

7.8 From Giulio Casserio and Odoardo Fialetti, *Tabulae Anatomicae* (Venice, 1627). Copperplate engraving. National Library of Medicine.

writings on the zombie's significance in contemporary culture—is on the potential of the living dead as a border crasher, whether this extends to politicized readings of the zombie as a stand-in for the immigrant and the refugee, or the microbe and virus's transversal of the epidermal walls that separate individual humans from their fellows and their environment. But his work also emphasizes the zombie *as* representation, replication, copy, in a way that is connected to the history of medical illustration. Much of Pfau's artistic experimentation in the zombie mythos is informed by an interest in how we represent the human pictorially in its most stripped-down version: for example, as living (vertical) or dead (horizontal). When is a form distinct as human rather than alien? When is a circle a head? And when is a severed head a human body part, an object of horror, or when is it, belonging to a zombie, merely a banal object in one's way? All of these issues relate to the questions that informed this study at the outset: when is a human body a person, and when is it, stripped, opened, subjected to the medical gaze, a thing?[11]

Of his medical illustrations, many of which incorporate the lowercase letter "I," Pfau (2013) says, "I'm very interested in the anthropomorphic quality of the lowercase and uppercase letter 'I.'" Indeed, looking at a series of thumbnails, I am struck by how often the form reappears, the singular personal pronoun like a stick man. The motif of the human outline recurs throughout Pfau's work, where he at times creates forms that resemble Keith Haring's people, and at others abstracts them further, as if he were trying to see what little economy of pencil strokes can still signify the human. At one point, he makes the word "ZOMBIE" itself into a form suggestive of the body. Like the stick figure, the zombie generalizes the specific, rendering the individual into a blank.

In Pfau's body of work, he often plays with how the human is visually represented and with different manners in which the most basic signifiers can suggest the zombie. In some renderings, the moment of contagion is represented, and the infected zombie is rendered in dotted line; it reaches out to touch another form and the dotted pattern begins to overtake other bodies. At other times, it is impossible to tell which figures are human and which are zombies: as with the corpses discussed in the previous section, the act of animation must come from outside.

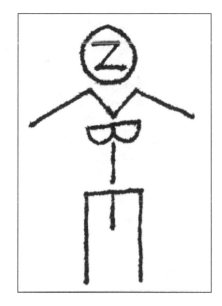

The illustration directly above (fig. 7.9), a close-up of one of Pfau's thin black line drawings, makes visible the way the ink bleeds into the paper, in keeping with the way Pfau's work continually emphasizes the blurriness of the human/nonhuman border. This is his intention even when the literal line is stark rather

7.9 George Pfau, "Zombieindex.us" (detail). Reprinted by permission of the artist.

than soggy. On this subject, Pfau (2014) has said, "One of my interests . . . is to appropriate the authoritative outlining/territorializing uses of the black line, in anatomy diagrams for example, and zombifying it, or poking holes in it, or showing its depth." As we've seen, Pfau's zombified medical models recall the way that some uses of the corpse inherently bend the line separating the living and the dead. More broadly, Pfau's illustrative experiments suggest, too, how the zombie narrative is itself a kind of floating signifier (much like that personal pronoun "I") capable of representing a range of contemporary concerns that culture reckons with—from fears of viral contamination, to racial prejudice, to anxiety about capitalism's abuses or the bleak, uncertain future of the planet's ecology. But, at its most basic level, Pfau's work suggests just how murky the dividing line is between the living and the dead, between the agentic "I" of subjecthood and the *objet petit* "i," if you will, of the inert thingness of the body.[12]

Live and Let Die?

In the series he calls "Trace," the silhouette that in Pfau's larger body of work becomes a motif, an oblique representation indistinguishable as either human or zombie, becomes the container for various human matter. Existing now only in the form of archival ink-jet prints of photographs taken of the original art objects, the ephemeral is underscored by the absent presence of these original objects. The series consists of four images, titled "Self Replacing Body Trace (Pores)," "Self Replacing Body Trace (Froth)," "Self Replacing Body Trace (Slough)," and "Self Replacing Body Trace (Meniscus)." In places, the human material used to create the form is recognizable: skin ("Pores"); hair and fingernails ("Slough"); at other times, less so. The titles "Froth" and "Meniscus," referring to the "curved upper surface of a column of liquid" (*Merriam-Webster*), may suggest the nature of the unidentified bodily fluids depicted therein, but more important, these "zoomed" works, like Pfau's close-up portraits of his oil paintings, suggest the difficulty of determining precise borders. This series emphasizes, in Pfau's (2014) words, the "subtle imprint we leave upon our surroundings"—that is, the microscopic traces of ourselves we shed as we move through the world, in skin cells, spittle, and dandruff. For Pfau (2014), this exploration relates to that place "where the illusion of 'self' hits a boundary or endpoint. If I were to lose an arm, is it no longer 'me'?" Similarly, on the micro level of the trace we are constantly dying; this facet of our existence—that we shed, slough, molt—suggests the inherent blurriness of vitality.

To me these images also make visible the way that absence is a presence, especially in the "Froth" piece, in which the humanoid silhouette is constituted in the negative space of a block of the foamy substance. The zombie is often identifiable not by its presence—the convention of appearing with graying, decayed flesh or red irises, let's remember, are relatively young updates to the genre—but by an act of subtraction, wherein only the difference between *what it was* and *what it is now* makes a body recognizable as a zombie. Pfau's work always reminds me that when we are talking about zombies (inasmuch as we are talking about histories of slavery and colonialism and the ravages of unchecked capitalism and toxic pollutants in our environment) we are also always considering the materiality of the corpse.

The fuzziness of Pfau's line—rendered literal in his zombiescapes, and perhaps rendered more figural in his medical illustrations—alludes to the fact that the parts we lose actually expand our borders and emphasize the uselessness of the fiction of the bounded, singular, agentic body, a central tenet of posthumanist explorations like those of Deleuze and Guattari. I've long accepted that one of the zombie's purposes is as a fetish that allows us to grapple with our being as living *assemblages* that consist always of both living and dead tissues: of human and nonhuman cells, of subject and object matter. Here, I've attempted to sketch out the zombie's usefulness as a model for considering the way we think about corpses as useful objects and, by extension, to gesture to the sometimes fuzzy line between cultivating respect for nonhuman entities and being aware of the dangers of considering human bodies not as people but as things.

To add another layer of complexity: though the corpse may be a Zombie Object, the zombie is not a corpse, but a broken corpse. Because it is animated it is a *broken* broken object: it isn't doing the thing it is meant to do—just lie there and work as the receptacle of our affect. Instead, animated by its own (or an alien) force, it defies our uses for the dead. The zombie is thus both a reflection of what we do to the corpse, making it our vehicle for a range of purposes or musings, and a resistance to that usurpation. Even this aspect of its being is in line with what I have elsewhere (Lauro 2015) termed "the zombie's dialectic": an irresolvable tension between imagery of servitude and of rebellion, a component of the zombie's makeup that is deeply tied to its colonial origins and its founding in Haiti, the site of the world's most famous slave revolt. What better model is there to suggest the utterly dire human condition than the zombie? For if we conceptualize the body as an object, we are both slaves to our bodies and their masters, until that ultimate moment when they thwart our best efforts to continue breathing.

What I've outlined in this study of the zombie art of George Pfau and its attention to the history of medical illustration—and in my articulation of the anatomical model as one type of Zombie Object—is not so much an ontology as a "(n)ontology." To me this means making room within our understanding of (our human) being for our interfaces with the nonliving thing, the nonexistent, and the things that are no longer there, of which the corpse is perhaps the most striking test case.

NOTES

1. The phenomenon of *Body Worlds* begins in the first years of the twenty-first century, and the number of exhibitions held globally are staggering. Its website boasts, "To date more than 40 million people throughout the world have visited *Body Worlds* exhibitions, making them the most successful traveling exhibitions of all time." See http://www.bodyworlds.com/en/exhibitions/past_exhibitions.html. See also Squier's (2004, 171–75) useful discussion of von Hagen's work.

2. For a critique of OOO, see Brown (2013).

3. Morton (2011, 151) clarifies: Since an object is withdrawn, even "from itself," it is a self-contradictory being. It is itself and not-itself, or in a slightly more expanded version, "There is a *rift between essence and appearance* within an object (as well as 'between' them)."

4. This constitutes a major difference between Heidegger and Harman. For Heidegger (1962, 67), "Handiness is the ontological categorical definition of beings as they are 'in themselves.'" For Harman, the Real Object (what we might imagine would be something like the object "in itself") can never be glimpsed, and the unhandiness (or presence-at-hand, or *Vorhandenheit*) of the broken tool merely *suggests* the existence of this inaccessible Real Object.

5. See Bryant (2010) for a discussion of flat ontology.

6. See Bennett (2010, 9) for discussion of Latour and Guattari. Bennett writes that Adorno "dares to affirm something like thing-power" (16), using her term for those moments in which objects "become vibrant things with a certain effectivity of their own" (xvi), but he doesn't go far enough for her taste. Adorno cautioned that we not "place the object on the orphaned royal throne once occupied by the subject. On that throne the object would be nothing but an idol" (Adorno 1983, 181; quoted in Bennett, 16).

7. See http://stemcell.stanford.edu/research.

8. "Zombieindex.us" was once profiled on the blog *io9*. See Newitz (2013).

9. Pfau (2013) has said, "Zombies provide us with a powerful lens into in-betweeness, recognition, contradiction, life and death, contagion, illness, otherness, appropriation/cannibalism, individuals and groups, colonialism, the body itself . . . my hope is that zombies can do more than just reinforce stereotypes and fears, and open up creative conversations about these things and many more . . . I'm hopeful about Mikhail Bakhtin's (and others') writing about the grotesque, and interested in bodily layering, and the mysterious unknown that lies beneath the skin, and is often feared or deemed 'ugly.' Why

must our grotesque oozing bits be stigmatized?"

10. Later anatomists, such as John Bell and William Hunter, would make it explicit that their models were cadavers, with Bell even often including the noose—as many anatomical subjects were executed by the state. See the Dream Anatomy Gallery of the US National Library of Medicine, http://www.nlm.nih.gov/dreamanatomy/da_g_I-D-1-15.html, which includes images of *Tabulae Anatomicae*.

11. I think here of the first medical illustration I remember seeing, William Hunter's 1774 engraving of a legless torso, with a fetus in utero nearly at term. The image is perhaps telling of the way many subvert the mother's role to merely that of a vehicle for her unborn child.

12. Here I am playing on the Lacanian *objet petit a*, which stands for "other," *autre*, signifying the unattainable object of desire. Perhaps *objet petit* "i" suggests *il-même*, a phrase that doesn't exist in French but by which we could signify the difference between the body itself and the person himself, *lui-même*.

REFERENCES

Adorno, Theodor W. 1983. *Negative Dialectics.* Translated by E. B. Ashton. New York: Continuum.

Ariès, Philippe. (1981) 2013. *The Hour of Our Death.* New York: Vintage Books.

Barnes, Djuna. (1915) 1994. *The Book of Repulsive Women: 8 Rhythms and 5 Drawings.* Los Angeles: Sun & Moon Press.

Bennett, Jane. 2010. *Vibrant Matter: A Political Ecology of Things.* Durham, NC: Duke University Press.

Brown, Bill. 2001. "Thing Theory." *Critical Inquiry* 28 (1): 1–22.

Brown, Nathan. 2013. "The Nadir of OOO: From Graham Harman's *Tool-Being* to Timothy Morton's *Realist Magic: Objects, Ontology, Causality.*" *Parrhesia* 17 (1): 62–71.

Bryant, Levi. 2010. "Flat Ontology." *Larval Subjects.* February 24. https://larvalsubjects.wordpress.com/2010/02/24/flat-ontology-2/.

Cohen, Jeffrey Jerome. 2014. "Grey." In *Prismatic Ecology: Ecotheory beyond Green*, edited by Jeffrey Jerome Cohen, 270–89. Minneapolis: University of Minnesota Press.

Deleuze, Gilles, and Félix Guattari. 1983. *Anti-Oedipus: Capitalism and Schizophrenia.* Translated by Brian Massumi. Minneapolis: University of Minnesota Press.

———. 2008. *A Thousand Plateaus: Capitalism and Schizophrenia.* Translated by Brian Massumi. London: Continuum.

Harman, Graham. 2002. *Tool-Being: Heidegger and the Metaphysics of Objects.* Peru, IL: Open Court.

———. 2011. *The Quadruple Object.* Washington, DC: Zero Books.

Heidegger, Martin. 1962. *Being and Time.* Translated by John Macquarrie and Edward Robinson. New York: Harper & Row.

———. 1968. *What Is a Thing?* Translated by W. B. Barton, Jr., and Vera Deutsch. Chicago: H. Regnery.

Lacan, Jacques. 1977. *Écrits: A Selection.* Translated by Alan Sheridan. New York: Norton.

Lauro, Sarah Juliet. 2015. *The Transatlantic Zombie: Slavery, Rebellion, and Living Death.* New Brunswick, NJ: Rutgers University Press.

Lauro, Sarah Juliet, and Karen Embry. 2008. "A Zombie Manifesto: The Nonhuman Condition in the Era of Advanced Capitalism." *boundary 2* 35 (1): 85–108.

Loechel, William E. 1960. "The History of Medical Illustration." *Bulletin of the Medical Library Association* 48 (2): 168–71.

Morton, Tim. 2011. "Objects as Temporary Autonomous Zones." *Continent* 1 (3): 149–55.

McAlister, Elizabeth. 2012. "Slaves, Cannibals, and Infected Hyper-Whites: The Race and Religion of Zombies." *Anthropological Quarterly* 85 (2): 457–86.

Newitz, Annalee. 2013. "This Interactive Painting Can Explain Why We Are Still Obsessed with Zombies." *io9*, March 5. http://io9.gizmodo.com/5988778/this -interactive-painting-can-explain-why -we-are-still-obsessed-with-zombies.

Pfau, George. 2013. "Exhibition Notes." http:// www.georgepfau.com/.

———. 2014. Personal e-mail correspondence.

Self, Will. 2014. "From Weeping Warts to Leprosy: The Gruesome Art of Medical Illustration." *The Guardian*, June 2. http://www.theguardian.com/artand design/2014/jun/02/sick-rose-gruesome -art-medical-illustration-will-self.

Squier, Susan M. 2004. *Liminal Lives: Imagining the Human at the Frontiers of Biomedicine*. Durham, NC: Duke University Press.

Stommel, Jesse. 2014. "The Loveliness of Decay: Rotting Flesh, Literary Matter, and Dead Media." *Journal of the Fantastic in the Arts* 25 (2–3): 332–36.

8.

OPEN UP A FEW
ZOMBIE BRAINS

Objectivity, Medical Visuality, and Brain Imaging in *The Zombie Autopsies*

Lorenzo Servitje

Like so many of the contemporary zombie narratives, Steven Schlozman's *The Zombie Autopsies* went viral. In 2011 the illustrated novel spread through media outlets to medical students, the general public, and, later, even academic conferences such as the Narrative Medicine Conference at King's College in 2013. There is a film currently in production, directed by George Romero (of *Night of the Living Dead* fame). The novel's popularity and numerous other appearances earned the assistant professor of psychiatry from Harvard a celebrity status among zombiephiles. Beyond its convincing biomedical theorizations about the etiology of a zombifying pathogen, the text raises relevant and timely critiques of neuroscience, brain imaging, and how objectivity rests on medicine's visual culture.

Why is this zombie narrative so popular? It certainly gained some form of legitimacy by originating from a medical professional, differentiating it from other zombie narratives. Schlozman's discussion of it on a national radio show elicited something akin to the panic caused by Orson Welles's 1938 radio performance of *The War of the Worlds*, albeit on a slightly less dramatic scale—he received a number of e-mails from concerned viewers, asking questions such as "What is the best medicine to treat a zombic infection?" (Schlozman 2013). Furthermore, Schlozman's insistence that his zombie narrative can do legitimate pedagogical work in terms of neuroscience certainly appealed to technophiles and everyday media consumers, as demonstrated by the circulation of stories about Schlozman on media outlets like *io9*, *U.S. News & World Report*, and PBS.

The novel and author's popularity aside, I suggest that in addition to teaching lessons in neurobiology, the novel speaks to the kind of cultural work the zombie is doing, as both a producer and a product of our contemporary healthscape. In this chapter I explore how *The Zombie Autopsies* modifies the epidemiological model of the zombie to fit with the older model of a passively controlled, animate body, moving on to reveal how the text problematizes simple notions of "life" and "death" with respect to medical rubrics. I consider the parasitological iteration of the zombie with respect to medical visuality to see what *The Zombie Autopsies* can tell us about how contemporary medical culture and rhetoric present the brain.

While the novel is not a comic or a graphic novel in the traditional sense, it is a productive contribution to the field of graphic medicine because it can be considered as a kind of "graphic text" or "sequential art" (McCloud 1994, 9). As a graphic medical narrative, *The Zombie Autopsies* draws on the history of medical illustration and medical epistemology by supplementing the textual narrative of zombie dissection with illustration and captioning. Its composition provides a productive counter-narrative to the increasing cultural capital of neuroscience as a bioinformaticized and visible discourse. More specifically, the text contends against the supposed objectivity of these technologies, by using the problematics of the researchers in the novel documenting their work to cognitively estrange contemporary neuroimaging. Ironically, through its fictionalized illustration and highly unreliable narrator, *The Zombie Autopsies* calls into question the normalizing discourses of brain imaging, a technology whose rhetoric conceals its simulated and, as Joseph Dumit (2004, 77–80) has suggested, its "algorithmic" construction. I draw on the work of Lorraine Daston and Peter Galison (2007) to suggest that the text speaks to medicine's historical origins in the form of anatomical illustration, subsequently challenging the objectivity of contemporary, digital visualizations of the brain. The way in which science and technology studies (STS) comes together with the illustrated novel gives us a new way to think about what the zombie signifies in contemporary biomedical and popular culture: the union of zombie narrative and image reveals how neuroscience has become a significant technoscientific system of thought in defining subjects as dead or alive, human or inhuman, normal or abnormal—ideological differentiations that have become obscured as culturally produced and hence naturalized.

Microbiology and the Birth of the Crypt

This text is about histology, about gross anatomy. In the narrative, the zombie apocalypse has changed the way medicine can be researched and practiced, not only due to the ever-present threat of zombies but also due to the actions humans have taken against them. Because of the use of nuclear weapons as an anti-epidemiological measure, digital technology has become unreliable: there are no computer models of the zombifying pathogen's misfolded protein, no useful digital infrastructure to communicate information from the lab to the WHO, and there is certainly no brain-imaging technology to explain how the brain of what the narrator and central medical organizations in the novel call "humanoids" can remain simultaneously deteriorated and functional. The imaging technologies are *not* there, and I am interested in thinking about why they are not there and what that tells us about their extant place in our world—a place where they *are* participating in "an epidemic of visualization" (Rose and Abi-Rached 2013, 74). Instead of brain imaging, the protagonists rely on pathological anatomy. In order to see how the disease works on the brain in real time, something they might be able to see in an fMRI or PET scan, for example, researchers must dissect the brains of undead subjects while these subjects remain "animate," writing down the results and drawing what they see.

The use of pathological anatomy with respect to medical knowledge and visuality suggests that the text provides a kind of "zombification" of Foucault's ([1973] 1994) "Open Up a Few Corpses." I say this in part to allude to Nikolas Rose and Joelle M. Abi-Rached's (2013, 56) development of the medical gaze to account for genomics, proteomics, and bioinformatics when they "pay homage to Foucault" by titling their section on imaging "Open Up a Few Brains." Schlozman's title also speaks to the zombification of that particular chapter of *The Birth of the Clinic* in a somewhat tongue-in-cheek capacity, as I would suggest that *The Zombie Autopsies* "reanimates" the earlier discourse of anatomical illustration and the understanding of life through death: defining life as the assemblage of functions that resist death (Buisson qtd. in Foucault [1973] 1994, 145), drawing from the nineteenth century anatomist Xavier Bichat, who, as Foucault argues, was one of the driving forces in the emergence of the medical gaze.[1] Dealing with the zombie in a medical framework brings us back to the medical confrontation with death, what gave "birth" to modern medical knowledge. Foucault notes it was pathological anatomy, the dissection of corpses soon after death to discover the how disease affected tissues, that changed medicine from a taxonomic system of disease classification to one where disease became localized inside and on the body of the patient. Bichat began to understand the concept of life by reverse engineering the process of death. Of those physicians who had not adopted the medical gaze, Bichat writes, "You have taken notes at patients' bedsides on affectations of the heart, the lungs, and the gastric viscera, and all is confusion for you in the symptoms, which refusing to yield up their meaning offer up an incoherent series of phenomena. Open up a few corpses: you will dissipate at once the darkness that observation alone could not dissipate" (qtd. in Foucault [1973] 1994, 146). The medical gaze was born in death, and to death medicine returns when investigating the zombie. With this new paradigm of medical knowledge, and subsequently professionalization, the patient begins to disappear and become his or her illness as clinicians "put the patient in parenthesis," in a way making them less than human and more objects of knowledge, an oft-cited critique of medical culture within the medical humanities.

This question regarding patients and objectification by the medical gaze becomes a pressing ethical dilemma in *The Zombie Autopsies*. Schlozman's novel is centered on the journal of Dr. Stanly Blum, a neurodevelopmental biologist working for the CDC, along with Dr. James Pitman, anatomist and medical illustrator. Blum and Pittman have been assigned to make a written record of the findings of Dr. Blanca Gutierrez, a microbiologist conducing humanity's last-ditch effort at understanding how the apocalyptic zombie pathogen functions, in order to create a vaccine. At this point, all of humanity is infected and the CDC predicts that humanity will cease to exist within a decade. They conduct research on an island site in the Indian Ocean, which the United Nations has labeled their Sanctuary and Study Site. The conditions of the research conducted on the island, however, contribute to the island being more commonly referred to as "The Crypt" because "those who volunteer to participate in the work on the island understand that return to [UN] bunkers is not permitted" (Schlozman and Sparacio 2011, 3), echoing a well-known character's speech from a popular zombie narrative: Rick Grimes's cathartic declaration "WE are the walking dead!" (Kirkman, Moore, and Adlard 2003–, issue 24).[2] The researchers become infected themselves and, in the case of Dr. Blanca Gutierrez, become research subjects once they progress to Stage IV of the disease—the point at which the WHO and the UN considers a person to be "ethically dead" and therefore a "humanoid" (Schlozman and Sparacio 2011, 168–70). In effect, they are all already dead.

"The Crypt" is a central thematic and titular referent: when Blum and Pittman arrive, they learn that the work is more anatomical than microbiological in nature—they are to perform dissections on the infected humanoids. While their charter claims that they are there to study molecular characteristics in addition to live zombies, only one of the images in the journal and a small percentage of the textual narrative display or discuss pathology at a molecular level. Neuromolecularization[3] has yielded the researchers no further understanding of how the disease operates beyond a level of identification that it is some kind of prion and influenza amalgam. Furthermore, Blum writes numerous times that they have to "go back to the beginning," that they "must have missed something" (Schlozman and Sparacio 2011, 31). The return to basic gross anatomy in the narrative runs parallel to the cultural work done by Schlozman's novel: it allows us cognitively to estrange, to defamiliarize technologies and definitions that have become black boxed and naturalized; that is, it borrows a mode from science fiction where the fictional, alternate reality of a text establishes a distance from our own reality so that we can see with it "fresh eyes" (Csicsery-Ronay 2008). To borrow Sarah Lauro's term from her essay in this volume, the text performs a kind of "overexposure."

One of the most highly regarded aspects of Schlozman's novel is that it is extensively biomedical. The book is in some capacity an extended theorization on the pathogenic effects and subsequent pathophysiological mechanisms that could make one a zombie. The zombie disease is not referred to as such; neither is it the ominous and generic "the Virus" or "the Infection," as is commonly seen in contemporary zombie narratives. Infected humans are not just suffering from one disease but a polyvalent infection, which causes the syndrome colloquially known as zombification, but is diagnosable as Ataxic Neurodegenerative Satiety Syndrome (ANSD) (Schlozman and Sparacio 2011, 3), a disease with a multifactorial etiology: more than one pathogen causes ANSD.

The microbiological pathophysiology draws on different strands of biomedical discourse that are enmeshed with zombie culture. The disease is transported by airborne droplets that carry a virus that is similar to seasonal influenza. This, of course, follows the paradigm that a virus engenders the zombie apocalypse, as in *28 Days Later* (Danny Boyle 2003) and countless other zombie narratives, in addition to speculations and iterations of zombie viruses in popular media and culture.[4] In the text, the body of the influenza-like virus contains prions, which are the central agents causing zombic symptoms. Prions, also known as proteinaceous infectious particles, alter normal versions of the proteins primarily related to central nervous system tissue, causing them to misfold into nonfunctional geometries,[5] making plaque-like formations called amyloids. They are the pathogens responsible for a number of neurodegenerative diseases such as Creutzfeldt-Jakob disease, fatal familial insomnia, and, most notoriously, bovine spongiform encephalopathy, more commonly known as mad cow disease, along with the cannibalism-borne Kuru.[6] Prion diseases resonate with Schlozman's text in terms of diagnosis: to definitively confirm the diagnosis of a prion disease usually requires an autopsy.[7] Furthermore, much like the way in which the zombie blurs the lines between life and death, prion disease continues to represent a challenge to biomedical research in that the exact mechanism by which prion disease causes cellular death in neurological tissue is still contested and, until the early 2000s, has remained under-researched. Prions, in effect, have remained resistant to the neuromolecular gaze. This connection between diagnostic techniques required in actual practice versus the only available mode of examination in the novel speak to the way the text asks us to question how certain "objective" medical truths come to be, namely, legal versus biological death and the diagnostic conclusions drawn from brain imaging.

Another connection between the novel and current biomedicine is the suggestion that the third pathogen is responsible for ANSD. As discussed in the introduction to this volume, there has been a rise in the popularity of using the zombie metaphor to explain and characterize insect and mammalian parasitology. Following the biomedicalization of the zombie in popular culture around the early 2000s, certain parasites that hijack host nervous systems and alter instinctual and conscious behavior have been termed "zombie parasites." *T. gondii* is especially relevant as it has been linked to altering human behavior, increasing risky activity, aggression, and suicidal ideation (Okusaga and Postolache 2012). These ideas of master-slave / host-parasite control are evocative of both the voodoo, "slave" zombie and of the infectious, medicalized model. Schlozman links these two zombie histories, or better, etiologies, through neuroscience.

As we are fascinated by all things neuro—such as the neurobehavioral implications of parasitology—Schlozman's pathophysiology is not only believable but also rhetorically convincing. More important, however, the use of prions and parasites with respect to the zombie demonstrates how the developments of neuroscience make it increasingly difficult to sustain certain binaries. Clear-cut boundaries in terms such as "life," "sick," "death," and even the "self"—if we think about the way microbes can affect behavior—are less black-and-white and, appropriately, more gray. This is particularly evident in the way the text deals with the bioethical questions surrounding the dissections.

Dissecting "Brain Death"

When Blum theorizes the way the disease works on a larger evolutionary scale, he suggests that "it broadens our biological niche at the expense of everything that makes us human," and finally comes to the conclusion that "humanoids are the hosts. They're the disease itself. Stage IV ANSD victims are the disease . . . *What does No Longer Human mean?*" (Schlozman and Sparacio 2011, 92). Bringing this back to the medical gaze, we could certainly read this as a kind hyperbolic objectification of patients: they become objects of knowledge, repositories for disease to be studied. Schlozman's novel offers a more nuanced critique of this operation, specifically in terms of the category of brain death and diagnosis with brain imaging.

How the disease becomes the host both biologically and nominally speaks to the bioethical questions that the text overtly raises: whether the dissections are vivisections or autopsies. The novel's peritextual material, the illustrations along with the appendixes that contain the UN's "Emergency Resolution Adopted by the General Assembly with Cooperation from the World Interfaith Council Pertaining to Status of Humans Suffering from Ataxic Neurodegenerative Satiety Deficiency Syndrome" (163), allows the medico-legal mode to redefine the concept of "human rights" based on those no longer able to "exercise the most basic human attributes that qualify for protection with respect to international guidelines" (Schlozman and Sparacio 2011, 165). To this effect, Blum goes out of his way to dehumanize subjects. Attuned to medical taxonomization and linguistic precision, Blum and the fictionalized international health organization are careful when characterizing their research as autopsy. One who is schooled in medical history might be quick to correct the author and the protagonist by suggesting that these are not autopsies but rather vivisections: they are, after all, incising and excavating a body which has "basic" brain function, respiration, heart rate, and metabolism. The implications of such questions speak to, among other things, the redefinition of death as brain death and the technical and legal questions surrounding this redefinition: namely, shutting off life support and harvesting organs for transplants. However, this is precisely the ethical issue at hand for the researchers and, by extension, the reader: zombies are legally dead, but are they dead biologically? These are not the kind of zombies that

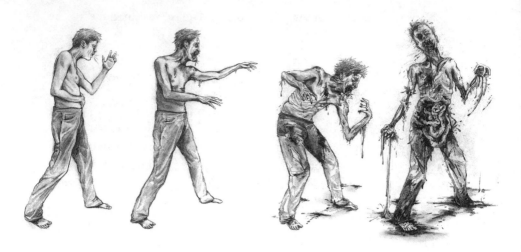

8.1 "Stage I—Stage II—Stage III—Stage IV." From *The Zombie Autopsies: Secret Notebooks from the Apocalypse* by Steven C. Schlozman, M.D. Illustrations by Andrea Sparacio. Copyright © 2011 by Steven C. Schlozman, M.D. Illustrations copyright © 2011 by Andrea Sparacio. Used by permission of Grand Central Publishing.

rise from the grave; they are people that have a neurological disorder who have progressed through to the fourth stage of the disease (fig. 8.1),[8] at which point the medical authorities diagnose them as "No Longer Human" (170), adeptly abbreviated as NLH. Language is critical here, as medical culture can define the rubrics that humanize or dehumanize, allowing for practices like "harvesting" to become acceptable. In Schlozman's novel, the illustrations not only reflect this reality but also put it into question. Take for instance the disease process narrated visually in stages.

Since the text is conveying both textually and graphically that life is defined by the function of certain parts of the brain, namely, the brain stem, the ethical questions the novel implies are indicative of bioethical arguments surrounding what constitutes death versus brain death—and subsequently what can be done with the bodies. Yet, while we get this information in the text, the figure above does not show us neurodegeneration—only its effects, and the intracranial images show us only those that have arrived at Stage IV. We are left to imagine the state between III and IV. The UN position on Stage IV (appendix 3) acknowledges that "neurologic changes that promote cognitive aggression and cannibalism in the absence of sound recognition of the moral inconsistences therein" qualify those at Stage IV as "NOT HUMAN" (Schlozman and Sparacio 2011, 169); consequently, "the protections afforded human and other biological subjects in the course of medical experimentations are not required for those with Stage IV ANSD" (170). This definition is followed by section 9, which states, "With regard to Medical Experiments it is acknowledged that I. Great Haste is necessary" and "II. Current neuro-biological evidence suggests a lack of somatosensory input, rendering such actions as general anesthesia unnecessary and time consuming" (170). The medico-legal construction of NLH / Stage IV is founded on necessity as well as scientific evidence, and, due to the state of the world in the text, the former takes precedence. Margaret Lock (2002) makes a similar suggestion with regard to the emergence of the notion of brain death or "the new death," what she argues is a medico-legal construction that was created for the purpose of facilitating organ transplantation.[9] Much like the zombie, the brain-dead patient dies twice.[10]

In contrast to the zombification of a medical student who harvests organs from a body that Michael Green, Daniel George, and Darryl Wilkinson discusses in their contribution to this volume, Blum is not worried about the person that is or was, but rather he is upset about the part of the brain that functions as an icon for the abstract notion of what constitutes humanity: "The frontal lobe makes us human, and its destruction robs us of our humanity" (Schlozman and Sparacio 2011, 46). Further fetishizing the frontal lobe, Blum writes, "For God's sake this is the frontal lobe. This is the higher brain, the human brain, the marvel of the known universe. It's the part of the brain that makes us wonder, makes us dream, makes us pray . . . I'm angry. I am looking at the frontal lobe and it's indistinguishable from decomposed matter" (54–55). The text deliberately foregrounds Blum's emotional state to question his judgment—he is angry at this decomposed matter. Similar to his own cognitive capacities, the very notions of humanity based on brain capacity and activity are decomposing and eluding his grasp, much like the rotted neocortex he holds in his hand.

We see this again even more prominently in another dissection scene where text and image work together to depict the breakdown of Blum's objectivity. Blum "removed the dermal layers, placing them over the eyes of the unconscious humanoid. . . . [If not] it will stare at its own beating heart with dead eye, and [he doesn't think he] can stand that incongruity" (Schlozman and Sparacio 2011, 86). What is interesting here is how this relates to real-world autopsy practice: namely, peeling back the scalp to expose the skull, allowing the skullcap to be removed with an oscillation saw. While necessary for excising the skullcap, the technique also covers the eyes and face, depersonalizing the cadaver. In the text, every single zombie image that includes the head has the eyes wide open—showing the incongruity that

Blum himself is able to deny in his writing but not in his drawings. The reader never gets this privilege. We are forced to bear witness to the seeming incongruity, facilitated by the interaction/conflict between image and text that opens a space for interrogation.

The zombies in this novel are, indeed, not zombies. Blum and the different medico-governmental apparatuses attempt to make that clear. They *are* "humanoids" who *were* "human" and *have* "died." But they are not "dead." Humanoids cannot die or live; they can only be animate or de-animate. In the spirit of good science fiction, this is not meant necessarily to make us question death and life or human and inhuman should there be a zombie apocalypse. Rather, this question of liminal humanity inculcates a cognitive estrangement that raises questions regarding the definitions of brain death both legally and biologically. Zombies reveal the way medical discursive constructs go beyond the general, binary rubrics of living and dead. This logic asks us to return to Bichat and Foucault and think about death less as the opposite of life, and instead to confront the way life and subjectivity are less "natural" than we would assume. As with the pressing apocalyptic pandemic in the narrative, these extreme circumstances reveal the way in which medical categories are not simply natural or inherently biological but are constructed by assemblages of people and systems of thought. This image/text interaction defamiliarizes the way different kinds of lives are built through neuroscience, specifically how identities are construed through scientific disciplines, technology, laws, and machines. The biomedical zombie in Schlozman's novel follows this logic to problematize the increasing neuropsychiatric definitions of normal and abnormal brains with the use of imaging.

Picturing Zombiehood

As the medical gaze has advanced into neuromolecularization, it has taken a different biopolitical and informatic turn. The gaze has shifted from Bichat's pathological anatomy to Rose's (2007, 70–71) "somatic self," which defines life based on molecular biological markers like genomics, a self predicated on developing neurochemical standards. Life is no longer that which resists death but rather that which most closely identifies with "the normal."[11] Rose shifts contemporary biopolitics from a "make live" and "let die" binary to a biopolitics of risk, where medical surveillance and disciplinary apparatuses are geared toward a model of normalization based on biology (91). Considering this notion of risk with respect to deviation from the normalized brain, the zombie in this text challenges the techniques by which this kind of biopolitical diagnostic operates.

Drawing inspiration from Sarah Juliet Lauro and Juliet Embry's (2008) "A Zombie Manifesto," I would suggest that the zombies in this text do not offer a solution to or an alternative from the subject/object divide, nor do they propose the possibility of hybridity that Haraway's cyborg offers. The zombie figure does not suggest that we should reject neuromolecular biology or brain imaging. Instead, the zombie crashes the system: both the digitalization of neuropsychiatric personhood on a material level—as imaging technologies do not work reliably—and the systems of thought that have engendered it as a biomedical technology. On a diegetic level, the zombies are the cause of the nuclear bombs that subsequently make digital technology unreliable. This etiology leads to an allegorical reading where the text asks us to question the assumptions and implications of digital brain imaging technologies with respect to what Joseph Dumit (2004) calls "picturing personhood."

The autopsies can be divided into to three categories: cranial, thoracic, and abdominal. This chapter primarily focuses on the images pertaining to the cranial, although it is worth noting that the excavations into the heart, lungs, and abdomen of the humanoids is contingent on the neurological correlative that keeps it functioning, namely, the possible parasite-like pathogen that protects the hypothalamus and brain stem. The objective is to discover the pathophysiology for ANSD. The brain stem remains intact, although the rest of the higher brain anatomy deteriorates along with its function, but something keeps the heart beating, the oxygen perfusing, and the nutrients metabolized to keep the humanoid animate, a process that baffles the investigators and readers.

The first illustration pertaining to the humanoid dissection (fig. 8.2) is perhaps the salient example of the text's allusion to medical illustration as a historical discourse preceding bio- and neuroinformatics because it draws on what is the one of the most iconic anatomical images in the history of medical illustration. This allusion primarily takes the form of the articulations of the neck: the head is rotated to the left and laterally flexed to a small degree again to the left; the cranium is sliced sagittally to reveal the inner structure. We can see anatomical positioning that is almost identical to one of the most well-known and circulated covers of *Gray's Anatomy* (fig. 8.3). Furthermore, the presence of restraints in many of the images recalls a technique and visual trope used by sixteenth-century anatomist Andrea Vesalius

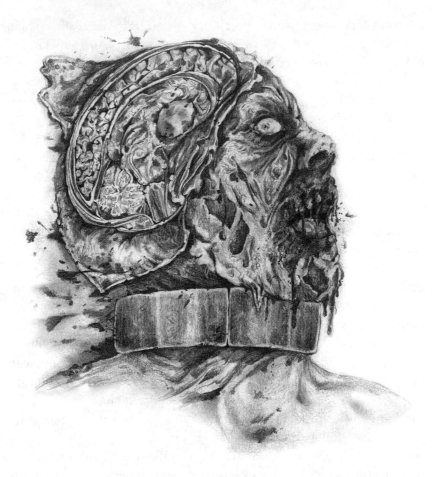

8.2 "Note the widened sulci suggesting profound cortical deterioration." From *The Zombie Autopsies: Secret Notebooks from the Apocalypse* by Steven C. Schlozman, M.D. Illustrations by Andrea Sparacio. Copyright © 2011 by Steven C. Schlozman, M.D. Illustrations copyright © 2011 by Andrea Sparacio. Used by permission of Grand Central Publishing.

in his *De Humani Corporis Fabrica* (1543), where the cadavers were held up by ropes, stakes, and other orthopedic devices. These kinds of allusions and historical residues highlight the overlap between art and science in medical visuality, which asks us to question our notions of objectivity. While this is not the case for all medical illustrations, in the eighteenth and early nineteenth century there was a visual-epistemic imperative that preceded this period to draw things not in their particular individuality but rather in reference to their ideal form. This technique aimed to achieve the best representative of the subject, what Daston and Galison (2007, 75) term "truth-

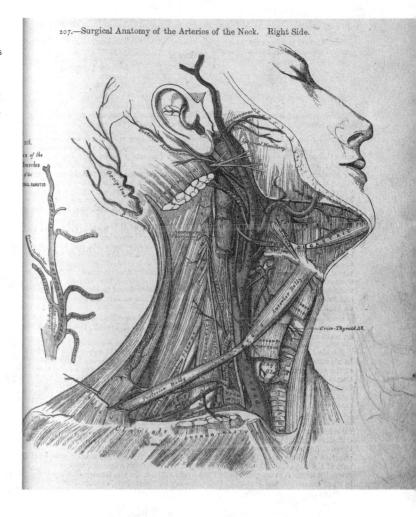

8.3 "Common Carotid: Surgical Anatomy of Arteries of the Neck. Right Side." From Henry Gray, *The Anatomy of the Human Body*, 2nd ed. (1860). Courtesy of King's College London, Foyle Special Collections Library.

to-nature." However, rather than using this as a critique of hand-drawn medical illustration, let me suggest that, in fact, this is a function of the text's critique of neuroimaging and its rhetoric of accuracy and objectivity.

Figure 8.2 draws on an older tradition of medical visuality, one that includes a complication of the subjectivity and objectivity of the artwork and the aura surrounding its production. While we have the older model of "truth-to-nature," where the illustrator and the anatomist—comparable to Blum working with Pittman—were consciously aware of the subjectivity imposed on their atlas, as they wanted to draw on their experiences to make an ideal image, the allusion to *Gray's Anatomy* makes the image more epistemically ambiguous. The shift from the idealized subjective imposition of the atlas maker into the idealized image shifted during the mid-Victorian period to a different model, what Daston and Galison (2007, 45) call "mechanical objectivity." In this model, those who created scientific images, of which many were reproductions from the microscope, valued restraint and the removal of themselves as much as possible from the creation of the image so that they could "let nature speak for itself." Practitioners of mechanical objectivity made it an imperative to intervene as little as possible, even going so far as to leave lens scratches and other artifacts of production in images. Atlas makers feared that they would impose their own theories onto the image and thereby skew its accuracy.

First published in 1858, *Gray's Anatomy*, written by Gray and illustrated by his colleague Henry Vandyke Carter, was produced during a transitional period between "truth-to-nature" and "mechanical objectivity." As Daston and Galison note, these shifts are not discrete and rigid, and so *Gray's Anatomy* both carries the illustrative resonances of earlier volumes like Vesalius's *Fabrica* and also consciously tries to remove the anatomists from the representations of the body. Gray, as an itemizer, remains opaque and reveals little about himself, assuming "the formal nondescript 'objectivity' of the authoritative medical man" (Richardson 2009, 15). Drawing on this history, the use of historical allusion in the form of blending image and text contributes to the critique of imaging technologies that are the products of a very different visual regime.

The first cranial panel, along with its textual narrative, clearly illustrates the conditions of its production: research imperatives; the questionable mechanical objectivity of the artist, Pitman (he has begun to show signs of progressive ANSD); and the problems with the "trained judgment" of the narrator, Blum (he is unpracticed in dissection and in encountering Stage IV humanoids, not to mention emotionally distraught). Furthermore, we are continually reminded of the unreliability of computers and other forms of digital media. This failure of digital technology brings to the surface the shift in the truth index of the visual and its relationship to objectivity. The researchers need to rely on handwritten notes and illustrations because "the computer infrastructure is too shaky" (Schlozman and Sparacio 2011, 25). Blum's repeated reference to the way they must make do without the use of many modern technologies depends on how the digital becomes, in many cases, a gold standard for accurate representation and transfer of information in both the medical community and popular understanding. At the same time, he acknowledges that, beyond the problems with electronic storage and transmission, digital media do not accurately capture the anatomy of the zombie, which follows the critiques made by STS and biomedical scholars that challenge the standard of objectivity in the digital.[12] Blum states that he has seen photographs of zombie anatomy before; however, he claims that "photographs don't tell the whole story. This stuff moves. The brain material literally changes shape as we expose it" (41).[13] It is as if Blum allegorizes a kind of "observer effect" in his object of study that parallels the way objective representation is not as untouched by human interference as it is thought to be.

Of course, text and illustration cannot tell the whole story. The novel's narrative is built around the questioning of reliability, where text and image attempt to validate each other; however, under the strains of succumbing to neurological effects of the disease, the abjection of the work, and the inability to use modern imaging and documentary technologies, the team still finds it difficult to "maintain the integrity of their investigation" (Schlozman and Sparacio 2011, 51). As they progress in their dissections and the stages of the disease, they have to try to "stay focused and detached" (46) and be "as objective as possible, to dispassionately include every detail" (52). Is Pittman drawing the humanoids as they are, or interjecting his own emotional despair and frustration, converting it into visual/textual monstrosity? Halfway through the text, Blum's handwritten notes are separated with a typed qualification: "Forensic psychologists and psychiatrists are confident that Blum's wandering train of thought, his dreams that almost sound like visions, are potentially the first signs of mental deterioration. *From this point forward, readers are advised to consider Blum's thoughts as neither clearly nor consistently coherent or objective*" (103). These problems are coupled with Blum's description of Pittman's degeneration into Stage IV right before his eyes. In this narrative of unreliability, the text challenges the production of biomedical knowledge as strictly objective in this specific context. However, this critique extends beyond the fictional world of the novel to the technological assemblages, specifically imaging, that we use in place of vivisecting patients.

Radiation is a critical artifact in the text. It is invisible yet it holds the plot with a death grip, circumscribing the kinds of knowledge that biomedicine is able to produce as "objective" understandings of the disease. The radiation from the nuclear weapons deployed by humans against the pathogen and zombies is what delimits the use of technology (Schlozman and Sparacio 2011, 73), what forces them to perform humanoid vivisections, what forces Blum to handwrite and Pittman to illustrate. In terms of neuroimaging, radiation can be read allegorically. If we use it as common topography to map *The Zombie Autopsies*, on one level, and the use of brain-imaging technologies, on the other, we can eliminate the possibility the text suggests that radiation is an imminent health hazard to our bodies in imaging technologies, although this is certainly a concern with repeated bouts of imaging. There is no reference to the radiation being a health hazard to the researchers or the medical teams off the island. The radiation causing the unreliability of digital technologies, in a self-referential fashion, gives us a way to pose a critique against brain imaging as a foundational mode of medical visuality whose reliability, precision, and accuracy are much more complicated than we, and even many medical professionals, might realize.

Joseph Dumit's (2004) work is helpful for understanding some of the complexities involved in characterizing the authenticity of brain scans. For the development of the technology an assemblage of professionals from various different disciplines—computer scientists, biochemists, physicists, nuclear pharmacologists, psychiatrists, and neurologists—must be mobilized and made to cooperate. Organic markers must be made into digital code, mathematically modeled, and then algorithmically converted into visual arrangements. Yet, despite these complexities, images are presented as "discrete, readable, and colorful . . . almost as simple as taking a snapshot" (57). The problem with complexity multiplies when we consider standardization and normalization of scans so that a differential diagnosis can be made. According to Dumit, these standardizations and normalizations are based on experiments, each with a number of stages, which include experiment design, measuring brain activity, making data comparable, and making data visible. Each stage, and its sub-steps, is hotly debated and plagued with assumptions about anatomy, physiology, and human nature (60). Furthermore, as Lisa Cartwright (1995, 23) has suggested, PET and MRI technologies can be traced back to disciplinary technologies like crainometers, calipers, and cephalometers used by nineteenth-century scientists to inscribe racial, sexual, and criminal difference in quantifiable forms. Thus brain imaging in its development and implementation is fundamentally entangled with the normalization of subjects. While each stage Dumit describes has its own problematics, for the purposes of this chapter I will refer only to problems with making data comparable and visible.

As a brain becomes digitized into numerical information representing radiotracer flow and as a result "apparent activation" (Dumit 2004, 81), to what is it compared to make a pathological determination? This process assumes a *generalized human brain*, which does not exist as such in the population. When determining what counts as brain activation in a particular area on a PET scan, the control—or average brain set—must be made from a sampling of brains. Statistical analysis and algorithms must be performed, such as subtraction and the averaging of brain set matrices, in order to determine diagnostic categories (81, 86). For example, if we wanted to define a schizophrenic brain, we would take a number of schizophrenic patient PET scans and average the data together; this set would then be subtracted from the average of "normal" patient scans and the resulting difference would be the data set for "the brain set of schizophrenia itself" (87). This speaks to the older visual-epistemic framework discussed above: these average brain sets are not creating a brain that exists in nature; rather, the algorithms are creating an "ideal" average to use as an atlas of comparison. Averaging is just one of the many decisions that have to be made to determine a reference image. For instance, there are also questions of threshold—how much brain activation is enough to light up the image? Dumit discusses these at length. There is little standardization across labs and imaging centers, which makes it difficult to transfer images out of their respective milieus, giving them a subjective quality particular to the network of actors that assemble their protocols and render their visualized form.

The Zombie Autopsies borrows the image/text combination from the comic book to render these questions visible. Suspending disbelief for a moment and ignoring the fact that Schlozman's novel is a fictional and massively reproduced piece, the sketches do retain an "aura," in the Benjaminian sense,[14] to the degree that they retain, albeit fictionally, the authenticity of the time and space of their production—the sketching of the autopsies as they were happening under these very subjective conditions, such as the lack of technological visualization and the neurological duress of the disease progression in both narrator and illustrator. This stands in contrast to imaging produced in laboratory scenarios. Rose and Abi-Rached (2013, 79–80) cite an example of the problematic conclusions drawn from fMRI studies where certain parts of the brain "light up" during a certain activity that is constructed in a lab scenario rather than in the "real world." In their function as simulations such images exemplify Daston and Galison's (2007, 383) fourth visual-scientific episteme: representation to presentation, following the paradigm of digital images that can be rotated, manipulated, correlated, and altered. Here the atlas makers are creating a kind of "engineering self" where the image is more tool than image, a presentation rather than representation. The function of presentation easily becomes a rhetorical tool, a problem that is evident in the way images are colored, altered,[15] and selected for inclusion in scientific publications, leading to a slippery slope when they become the basis for diagnostics. They are supplements to further an argument, rather than reflections of a reality in nature. In simulations like brain imaging, color is a clear example of an artifact that does not reflect nature but is instead a constructed value for presentation, a process Dumit (2004, 83, 90–94) explores at length.[16]

In terms of PET scans, we can consider what is essentially a black boxing of the complexity of the PET scan's *construction* of rendered brain images to be similar to the example of the fMRI simulation. These brain images lack the uniqueness of time and space; the context in which they were constructed is erased. If something like fMRI or PET is supposed to measure the neurological response to certain situations or certain images, how does one include the situation in the reproduction of the brain images? I take authenticity in this sense to mean it does not authentically reproduce the precise conditions of its production, something that the interaction between the illustrations of *The Zombie Autopsies* and their textual narrative brings to our attention. In this sense, the novel performs one of the disciplinary aims of graphic medicine—"disrupting the 'objective case study'" (Czerwiec et al. 2015, 3).

Schlozman's illustrated novel does not go so far as to suggest that we are "zombified" through the technological/biological determinism that the "epidemic" of brain visualization can impose in its norming functions. Yet, like the zombie, it avoids giving us clear-cut binaries. Schlozman's novel and its interplay between text and image draw our awareness to the construction of neuroimaging and the subsequent implications for how we define normal and pathological in our increasingly neuromolecular age—how, in a broader context, there has been an increasing "cultural move to visualize identity" (Joyce 2010, 198). Furthermore, like so many zombie narratives, it questions life and death but does so in a nuanced and productive fashion, by problematizing the specific notion of brain death. Utilizing medical illustration along with textual narrative, *The Zombie Autopsies* performs the work of graphic medicine in a way that appeals to the biology major as much as to the zombiephile.

NOTES

1. Cf. *"life is the totality of those functions which resist death"* (Bichat 1809, 1; emphasis in original).
2. See also Canavan (2010, 50).
3. The increasing understanding of the brain on a molecular scale. See Rose and Abi-Rached (2013).
4. The airborne trope is consistent with some popular theories and speculations about a real "rage virus" (to use the name of the zombifying pathogen in *28 Days Later*) emerging from a hybrid between influenza and rabies (Than 2013).
5. The treatment protocol in place induces metabolic alkalosis with sodium bicarbonate in conjunction with a diuretic, which is meant to slow the rate of prion propagation and misfolding.
6. Besides being responsible for progressive neurodegenerative symptoms that would be conducive to zombiism, such as impaired gait and cognitive capacities, prions are linked to a Kuru, which has a kind of intertextual relationship to diseases in zombie narratives. Endemic to highland tribal regions of New Guinea, Kuru causes cerebral and cerebellar damage leading to problems with gait (ataxia) and loss of speech and cognitive function. More significant is the vector of transmission. The disease spreads through the practice of funeral cannibalism: families of the deceased eat the highly infectious brain tissue of the dead. This, of course, resonates with the general zombic trope of cannibalism and the B-movie trope of groaning undead uttering only one intelligible phrase: "Brains . . . Brains. . . ." Schlozman re-creates this in a less dramatic, more clinical fashion when Blum notes that subjects prefer

central nervous system tissue and configures the "real-life" proteinaceous edible vector of transmission into an airborne form.

7. There have been recent tests developed that can aid this diagnosis. Imaging and cerebrospinal fluid can detect the disease to a high probability, and brain biopsy is sometimes an option, but the gold standard remains viewing the brain after death (Greenwood et al. 2012, 609).
8. The original illustrated novel contains captions in a font that mimics handwriting; however, these were not reproduced in the images provided, and thus are replicated textually rather than graphically.
9. See also "A Definition of Irreversible Coma" (1968).
10. For an extended reading and history of zombies vis-à-vis brain death see Luckhurst (2015).
11. For a more generalized theorization and oft-cited critique, see Canguilhem (1989).
12. See Dumit (2004) and Daston and Galison (2007). For a more recent critique within the discipline of pathology itself, see Tadrous (2010).
13. These are presumably digital photographs given the contemporary time period and the fact that he speaks to information being transferred from the site through telecommunications.
14. See Benjamin (2008). For the early media theorist Walter Benjamin, the aura of a work of art is its uniqueness in terms of the time, place, and conditions of its production. These qualities are not transferred when a piece of art is reproduced.
15. For a critique of current standards in scientific publication and attempted remedies, see Frow (2012).
16. See also Daston and Galison (2007, 413).

REFERENCES

Benjamin, Walter. 2008. *The Work of Art in the Age of Its Technological Reproducibility,* *and Other Writings on Media.* Edited by Michael W. Jennings, Brigid Doherty, and Thomas Y. Levin. Cambridge, MA: Belknap Press of Harvard University Press.

Bichat, Xavier. 1809. *Physiological Researches upon Life and Death*. Translated by Tobias Watkins. 1st US ed. from the 2nd French ed. Philadelphia: Smith & Maxwell.

Canavan, Gerry. 2010. "'We Are the Walking Dead': Race, Time, and Survival in Zombie Narrative." *Extrapolation* 51 (3): 431–53.

Canguilhem, Georges. 1989. *The Normal and the Pathological*. Translated by Carolyn R. Fawcett. New York: Zone Books.

Cartwright, Lisa. 1995. *Screening the Body: Tracing Medicine's Visual Culture*. Minneapolis: University of Minnesota Press.

Csicsery-Ronay, Istvan. 2008. *The Seven Beauties of Science Fiction*. Middletown, CT: Wesleyan University Press.

Czerwiec, MK, Michael Green, Ian Williams, Susan M. Squier, Kimberly Myers, and Scott Smith. 2015. *Graphic Medicine Manifesto*. University Park: Pennsylvania State University Press.

Daston, Lorraine, and Peter Galison. 2007. *Objectivity*. New York: Zone Books.

"A Definition of Irreversible Coma: Report of the Ad Hoc Committee of the Harvard Medical School to Examine the Definition of Brain Death." 1968. *Journal of the American Medical Association* 205 (6): 337–40.

Dumit, Joseph. 2004. *Picturing Personhood: Brain Scans and Biomedical Identity*. Princeton, NJ: Princeton University Press.

Foucault, Michel. (1973) 1994. *The Birth of the Clinic: An Archaeology of Medical Perception*. Translated by A. M. Sheridan Smith. New York: Vintage Books.

Frow, Emma K. 2012. "Drawing a Line: Setting Guidelines for Digital Image Processing in Scientific Journal Articles." *Social Studies of Science* 42 (3): 369–92.

Greenwood, David, Mark Barer, Richard Slack, and Will Irving. 2012. *Medical Microbiology*. Edinburgh: Churchill Livingstone.

Joyce, Kelly. 2010. "The Body as Image: An Examination of the Economic and Political Dynamics of Magnetic Resonance Imaging and the Construction of Difference." In *Biomedicalization: Technoscience, Health, and Illness in the U.S.*, edited by Laura Mamo, Adele E. Clarke, Jennifer Ruth Fosket, Jennifer R. Fishman, and Janet K. Shim, 197–217. Durham, NC: Duke University Press.

Kirkman, Robert, Tony Moore, and Charlie Adlard. 2003–. *The Walking Dead*. Comic book series. Berkeley, CA: Image Comics.

Lauro, Sarah Juliet, and Karen Embry. 2008. "A Zombie Manifesto: The Nonhuman Condition in the Era of Advanced Capitalism." *boundary 2* 35 (1): 85–108.

Lock, Margaret M. 2002. *Twice Dead: Organ Transplants and the Reinvention of Death*. Berkeley: University of California Press.

Luckhurst, Roger. 2015. *Zombies: A Cultural History*. London: Reaktion Books.

McCloud, Scott. 1994. *Understanding Comics: The Invisible Art*. New York: Harper Perennial.

Okusaga, Olaoluwa, and Teodor T. Postolache. 2012. "*Toxoplasma gondii*, the Immune System, and Suicidal Behavior." In *The Neurobiological Basis of Suicide*, edited by Yogesh Dwivedi, 381–407. Boca Raton, FL: CRC Press.

Richardson, Ruth. 2009. *The Making of Mr. Gray's Anatomy: Bodies, Books, Fortune, Fame*. New York: Oxford University Press.

Rose, Nikolas S. 2007. *Politics of Life Itself: Biomedicine, Power, and Subjectivity in the Twenty-First Century*. Princeton, NJ: Princeton University Press.

Rose, Nikolas S., and Joelle M. Abi-Rached. 2013. *Neuro: The New Brain Sciences and the Management of the Mind*.

Princeton, NJ: Princeton University Press.

Schlozman, Steven. 2013. "The Harvard Doctor Who Accidentally Unleashed a Zombie Invasion." *New York Times Magazine*, October 25. http://www.nytimes.com/2013/10/27/magazine/the-harvard-doctor-who-accidentally-unleashed-a-zombie-invasion.html.

Schlozman, Steven C., and Andrea Sparacio. 2011. *The Zombie Autopsies: Secret Notebooks from the Apocalypse*. New York: Grand Central Publishing.

Tadrous, Paul J. 2010. "On the Concept of Objectivity in Digital Image Analysis in Pathology." *Pathology* 42 (3): 207–11.

Than, Ker. 2010. "'Zombie Virus' Possible via Rabies-Flu Hybrid?" *National Geographic News*, October 27. http://news.nationalgeographic.com/news/2010/10/1001027-rabies-influenza-zombie-virus-science/.

9.

THE ANOREXIC AS ZOMBIE WITNESS

Illness and Recovery in Katie Green's *Lighter Than My Shadow*

Dan Smith

From Autobiography to Zombie Narrative

In Katie Green's *Lighter Than My Shadow* (2013), a five-hundred-page autobiographical graphic novel that addresses living with anorexia, the act of drawing and the creation of a graphic *herstory* facilitate a sense of agency, empathy, and an ongoing process of recovery. This is a realization of the task of witnessing. This witnessing occurs from a position that is outside the normative boundaries of embodied life, from the position of the zombie. There are no explicit references to the figure of the zombie in *Lighter Than My Shadow*, but nevertheless I would like to argue that, as well as operating as a work of graphic medicine, it becomes a zombie narrative. It is not an intentional authorial inscription in the work, but rather an emergent association, albeit one that sits outside familiar frameworks of genre and convention.

Todd Platts (2013, 549) historicizes the zombie as a (specifically North American) horror trope within the context of older folkloric traditions entering "the U.S. popular cultural imagination as a result of its military occupation of Haiti (1915–1934)." In their modern form, mainstream zombie narratives tend to present images of desolation and "apocalyptic parables" (547) of collapsed societies and groups of struggling survivors. *Lighter Than My Shadow* does not correspond to such traditions. The model of the zombie is also distinct from the more recognizable variety, an example of which is provided by Mathias Clasen (2010, 1): "an undead person—it could be your colleague, your neighbor, your grandmother—whose sole purpose is to eat you, alive." However, what we can recognize from Clasen's account is the concept of a blurring of distinction between life and death, and the fear of the zombie being a person close to you. Clasen describes zombies as violating "our intuitive understanding of death as the cessation of self-propelled motion and agency, as well as death as an irreversible event" (4).

The figure of the zombie evoked in *Lighter Than My Shadow* is not a monster in the conventional sense, but a protagonist pushed to the limits of subjectivity, perhaps even beyond the category of being alive. In this sense, the book resonates with recent sympathetic depictions of zombies, such as the French television series *Les Revenants* (*The Returned*) (2012—), based on a 2004 film of the same name; the BBC television series *In the Flesh* (2013–14); and the films *Life after Beth* (Jeff Baena 2014) and *Warm Bodies* (Jonathan Levine 2013). Kyle William Bishop (2010, 205) discusses this as a move toward depicting zombies as "sympathetic victims" (205), offering an example in the domestication of a zombie, formerly a principal character, in the film *Shaun of the Dead* (Edgar Wright 2004). In these examples, the zombie becomes monstrous in that it becomes an uncanny distortion of humanity. The apparent stability and centrality of the human is undermined. The character of Katie is shown approaching this threshold, the point from which she cannot return.

Green makes use of her medium to show us how Katie saw herself. In a sequence that allows us to view Katie viewing her own body, the top three panels of a page (Green 2013, 118) show Katie undressing down to her underwear and offering glimpses of how excessive her malnourishment has become. The reflections are not what we see when we look at her drawn body. Below, across two panels, Katie's body is contrasted with how she perceives her own reflection, shown as extreme magnifications of small body parts. Her thigh and belly are squished and squeezed, her flesh appearing grotesque and enormous in the mirror, framed by the dark of a black cloud that haunts Green's narrative.

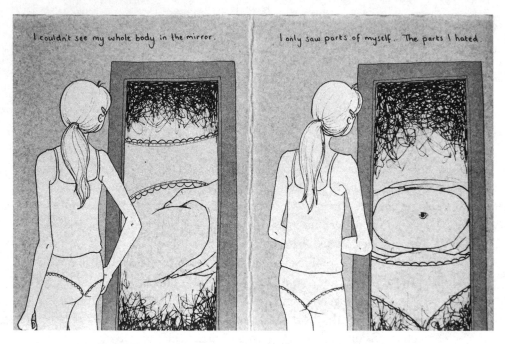

9.1 From *Lighter Than My Shadow* by Katie Green, published by Jonathan Cape. Reproduced by permission of The Random House Group Ltd.

The cloud then leaves the mirror as she moves to her bed, following her, surrounding her: "There was no escape from the thoughts . . . even when I slept" (119). Cakes and desserts, framed by the black cloud, populate her dreams and her body swells to obese proportions. When she is awake we see her showering, as if under a rainstorm coming from the cloud, her hands pulling loose clumps of hair from her head.

These images allow us to see what young Katie cannot and reveal, as her weight loss accelerates, how close she came to a barely human condition, her body closer to death than life, unable to act as a witness. The idea of the zombie here is as a physical and psychic condition of bodily emaciation and loss of agency. I would like to consider the figure of the zombie not through the tropes of horror but rather in terms of transformations of the human body—specifically, the possibility of transforming bodies into the conditions of the *Muselmann*, as discussed by Primo Levi, Maurice Blanchot, and Giorgio Agamben. Agamben's *Remnants of Auschwitz* (2002), a work that builds on the writings of Levi and Blanchot, addresses the embodied limitations of human life and the limitations of the idea of the witness. *Remnants of Auschwitz*, the third part of Agamben's *Homo Sacer* series, offers a rethinking of

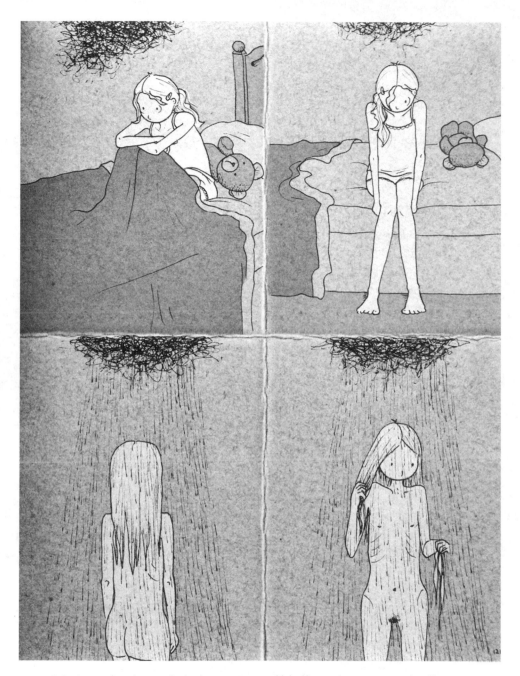

9.2 From *Lighter Than My Shadow* by Katie Green, published by Jonathan Cape. Reproduced by permission of The Random House Group Ltd.

ethics through considering acts of witnessing. The central issue of testimony, or rather of the untestifiable, is embodied in the figure of the witness who can be dead, yet not. The name of this dead / not dead figure, born out of a jargon of the camp, is *der Muselmann*. This was what the prisoners feared becoming, a state of physical and mental degeneration that rendered the subject closer to death than to life, exorcising sentience, agency, and subjectivity until all that appeared to remain were the properties of an animated corpse.

These uncanny dimensions of the Muselmann are echoed by Green's story of illness, of diminished physique and a body drained of life by trauma and breakdown in illness. This physical and psychic condition is a limit of life itself in terms of both subjectivity and how it is viewed as the Other. The Muselmann might be viewed as the nonfictional precedent of the zombie as it emerged in horror comics in the early 1950s. The Muselmann is already on the way to death. It is a boundary of ethics, a limit of the possibility of ethics. To be clear, my intention here is not to trivialize the Muselmann through comparison with a trope from popular culture, or to generate a potentially insulting equivalence of the Holocaust with anorexia or between sufferers of anorexia and zombies. Rather, I seek to illuminate a sequence of informative resonances, brought together in a graphic novel, regarding witnessing and extreme conditions of bodily experience and subjectivity. This intended reading can be thought of in terms of Susan Sontag's (1991) critical accounts of metaphor. In considering interpretations and articulations of illness, Sontag offers a resonant and powerful set of reflections on forms of metaphor that generate negative impact. She argues that metaphor encourages the generation of taboos and misinformation, which contribute to an overall negative impact on public perceptions of illness. However, rather than directly perpetuate the "lurid metaphors" (3) that Sontag identifies, I read Green's narrative visualization as a working against misinformation and negative perceptions. There is a mobilization of metaphorical elements at work that is active, reflexive, and empathetic. My introduction of the zombie as an additional layer of metaphor is intended to further describe and navigate this representational space.

The Zombie as a Witness

A resonant affinity between *Lighter Than My Shadow* and Agamben's *Remnants of Auschwitz* is the destabilizing of the witness. The idea of a witness is made problematic while, at the same time, attention is drawn to the importance and centrality of such figures, however unreliable their observations may be. In *Remnants of Auschwitz* the theorizing of language and alterity follows a lineage of thought, finding its direct precedent in the work of Maurice Blanchot's *The Writing of the Disaster* (1995). For Blanchot, writing is a condition in which the very thing it describes or represents is obscured by the act itself. Writing takes the place of the real. The disaster, a term used by Blanchot to describe the Holocaust, is similarly distanced, something we cannot experience, an experience we cannot understand (120). Language cannot represent the extreme conditions of the camps or convey what people went through there. Writing can stand in for this, but it is not this.

It is on such elusive yet poignant investigations of language and action that Agamben builds his own account. In *Remnants of Auschwitz* he looks to a space between explanation and mystification to engage with the ethics of witnessing. There is no constancy in either subjects or objects. We cannot know them or ourselves for certain. This lack of certainty brings into question the value of a statement made by the witness, destabilizes the primacy of acts of witnessing. For Agamben (2002) it is the Holocaust that occupies the central territory in the witness discussion. In the camp, he writes, "one of the reasons that can drive a prisoner to survive is the idea of becoming a witness" (15). Levi acts as an example for Agamben; he "tirelessly recounts his experience to everyone. He becomes like Coleridge's Ancient Mariner" (16). Levi's memories of imprisonment are more vivid than anything before or since, with acoustic and visual memories likened to being both etched in his memory and recorded on magnetic tape in preparation for bearing witness (27). However, testimony is problematic. Auschwitz must not be granted the mystical status of being unsayable, yet it is problematized by the question of testimony, which contains a lacuna. Survivors are not witnesses. Those who have not lived through it cannot know. Those who have will not tell. This lacuna "calls into question the very meaning of testimony and, along with it, the identity and reliability of the witnesses" (33). Central to Agamben's approach to understanding the Holocaust is the difficulty in understanding the witness and the possibility of witnessing. This is reflected in *Lighter Than My Shadow* in the refusal to reduce illness to something that can be accounted for simply and directly, which can be explained away with a simple cause. Rather, it is approached as something that by necessity is difficult to understand.

The Holocaust must be approached as something difficult to understand in order to ensure that it remains in the category of the impossible rather than the possible. There is as much danger in understanding it too quickly as there is in avoiding understanding altogether. Agamben does not attempt to resolve this problem, but seems to locate a specific inquiry into witnessing somewhere between these two negative tendencies. The Holocaust is an unrepresentable trauma. It offers a point of specificity yet becomes a general condition that forever transforms and redefines Western culture. The figure of the witness in relation to the Holocaust binds representation to ethics, not just in interpreting texts but also in terms of the task of philosophy, the structuring of new forms of politics and possibility through testimony. These qualities can be considered as potential forces at work in *Lighter Than My Shadow*. There is a tension between the specific autobiographical narrative and more general conditions of subjectivity, between unrepresentable forms and forms of representation, and between empathic understanding and the impossibility of understanding. *Lighter Than My Shadow* resists straightforward attempts at understanding in favor of an ethical bond between reader and author/protagonist.

Eric Cazdyn (2012, 8) places Agamben within a context of four concepts that have been mobilized to rethink global capitalism in terms of the colonization of life and death: "These are Slavoj Žižek's concept of the 'undead,' Jean-Luc Nancy's 'living dead,' Giorgio Agamben's 'bare life,' and Margaret Lock's 'twice dead.'" This accumulated rethinking of contemporary capitalism understands crisis as a condition that is not generated by things going wrong but that occurs when things go right (2). At the level of the subject, this is useful for understanding Katie's condition. Her anorexia develops through normative conditions, within middle-class domesticity, framed by conditions of contemporary Western capitalism. Her depiction of her memories of childhood offers a happy and stable context. However, the broader context here, for Cazdyn, is one of colonization, of healthcare as an industrial system of managing symptoms, while capitalism itself is a terminal condition, where the idea of a cure appears beyond the limits of cognition and imagination. Capitalism is a terminal condition that determines spaces of illness and representation more broadly. As sufferers of capitalism, subjects are already dead but are managed, treated indefinitely, as the diabetic is treated with insulin (2).

Lighter Than My Shadow is a reflection of illness from a perspective where things are closer to a normative state, created when the patient is functioning well. We read through situations that may well be terminal, haunted by the idea of fading away into oblivion, but from which we know there will come a chronic and ongoing process of redemptive survival: "The paradigmatic condition illustrating the already dead is that of the medical patient who has been diagnosed with terminal disease only to live through medical advances that then turn the terminal illness into a chronic one. The disease remains life threatening, still incurable, even though it is managed and controlled, perhaps indefinitely" (Cazdyn 2012, 4). Katie's disease remains life threatening and uncured, but must be managed indefinitely. The patient is afforded something that functions "like a hole in time" (Cazdyn 2012, 4), an escape route or trap door. However, for Cazdyn, this is an unbearable condition at the level of the social, which needs to be transformed. When considering the situation of Katie, the space of revolution is in the writing, in the transformation of the condition of the sufferer to the condition of writer or creator. For Cazdyn, recognizing the condition of the already dead is a means to rethink distinctions between life and death.

By recasting *Lighter Than My Shadow* as a zombie narrative, through Agamben's reading of the Muselmann, the narrative experience can be grasped and moved beyond the limiting frameworks of the management and stabilizing of the normative subject, and can illuminate unstable notions of change, subjectivity, and representations of illness. Rethinking death as an everyday presence is, according to Cazdyn (2012, 7), an engagement with ideological rhetoric, and a renegotiation of death as a form necessary for imagining radical change within social fields. Cazdyn's use of Agamben's ideas focuses on bare life, read as legally dead while biologically still living. This is a condition made possible by the denial of rights granted to the living, to former subjects who are forced into a zone between life and death, becoming nothing but bare life, for which the victim of Nazi concentration camps is the archetypal figure. Totalitarianism and democracy share this figure of life exposed to the terror of death as an originary form of relation, binding life with law, becoming more dominant as a structural principle over time until the exception becomes the rule. This is a structural order that is present both in the extreme conditions of Guantanamo and in contemporary medical practices.

The issue of witnessing offers a harrowing form in which we can recognize the disturbing realization of a key principle in Agamben's political thought: if power is able to construct and order the subject, it is also able to do the reverse, to disintegrate the subject. The central issue of testimony, of the untestifiable, is embodied in the figure of the witness who can be dead, yet not: *der Muselmann.* They are a boundary of ethics, a limit of the possibility of ethics. This name is highly problematic for contemporary readers, as the literal meaning is "the Muslim." The term *Muselmann* was commonly used at Auschwitz, and Agamben (1995, 45) takes the position that the most probable and convincing explanation is that the term was used as an application of the most literal meaning of Muslim as an Arabic word: "one who submits unconditionally to the will of God." The term reflects a European perception of Islam as fatalistic, that the Muslim is resigned to the conviction that the will of Allah is working within every event and action. The walking dead of Auschwitz were viewed as having lost the will to survive, to have submitted to an unconditional fatalism. For the inmates of Auschwitz, the proto-zombie could do nothing directly to harm you, but it was you who would end up like one. The zombie is conveniently dead. The actuality of the Muselmann is so much worse.

Embodiment and Illness

Lighter Than My Shadow is a work of daunting scale. The difficulty involved in creating a five-hundred-page autobiographical comic addressing growing up with anorexia is made explicit by the author: "Twelve years in the making from idea to publication, it is quite possibly the hardest thing I've ever done (and that's not discounting the story contained within the book itself)" (Green 2014). The narrative is one of illness and recovery, offering readers an empathetic encounter in a space of painful memories, shaped in words and pictures. We encounter Katie as a young girl, growing up in what seems a stable, loving environment. Katie's parents are kind, attentive, understanding, and patient. Yet it is not enough; the causal elements of Katie's illness may be social, and we read of the exacerbation of anxiety in the form of peer pressure, but this is not a story of blaming the home environment, of locating the roots of illness.

Her eating disorder is placed within a broader context of anxiety, a need for control, and opens Katie up to ongoing exploitation and sexual abuse. An adult Katie is depicted working on the book, reflecting on what she thinks were the signs of an eating disorder taking hold; she considers why nobody noticed the signs and concludes that there was no reason to, as her memories are of being happy. A page without panel separations shows Katie and her sister playing together outside: "My childhood was perfect. I never wanted it to end" (Green 2013, 37).

The absence of panels suggests an unbroken and undefined duration, without the boundaries of either diegetic or readerly temporality. The only temporal boundaries are that of the page and of the inevitability that the

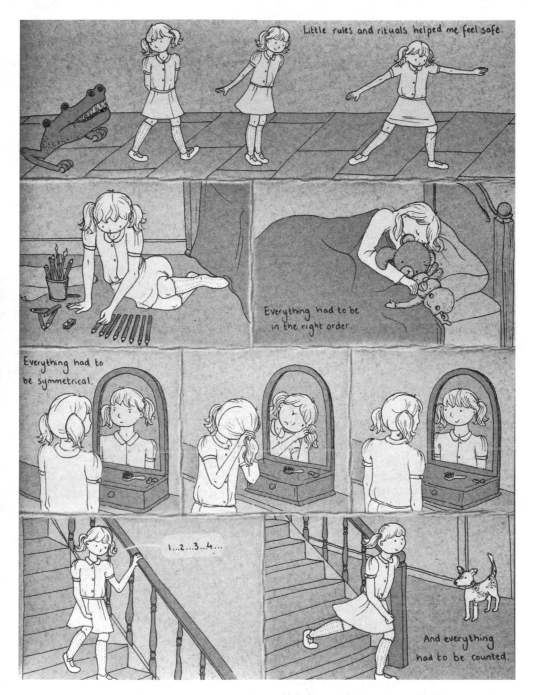

9.3 From *Lighter Than My Shadow* by Katie Green, published by Jonathan Cape. Reproduced by permission of The Random House Group Ltd.

depicted period of childhood and play must have ended. The following pages, despite a subtle shift in the use of color and the return to panel divisions, show Katie as equally happy with her best friend, Megan (Green 2013, 38–39). Each page is drawn using outlines in black, with some tonal areas, each variations of a set of soft hues, resembling pastel-colored sheets of paper. The panel borders are not hard black lines but comprise fold marks, as if the paper has been doubled over and creased along an edge. These formal devices generate a subtle intimacy, bringing the reader closer to the narrative world Green creates and intensifying the emotional and empathetic possibilities of reading encounters. These formal elements can also be read as identifying with a handmade and childlike set of materials and qualitative associations. The colors resemble scrapbook pages or sketchbooks of pastel tones. The folding and creasing, suggestive of making do by hand, together with the style of drawing, deceptively simple, convey associations of naïveté and innocence, work toward a contrived sense of making reality softer, perhaps even sentimental or cute. In addition to achieving what Scott McCloud (1994, 30) calls "amplification through simplification," the design and drawing reflects the general position described by Elisabeth El Refaie (2012) in her book *Autobiographical Comics: Life Writing in Pictures*, in which she observes that many autobiographical comics have resisted the appearance of realism in favor of forms of stylized estrangement.

I would like to suggest that Green's formal and stylistic decisions are more particular, connecting adult reflection to an imagined world of childhood, a tension that has been identified as a significant presence within accounts of anorexia. In particular, childhood and the softness of approach contribute to an unsettling atmosphere around *Lighter Than My Shadow* that corresponds to Fredrik Svenaeus's (2013) research into anorexia and his application of ideas related to the uncanny. The happy home is presented as a form of uncanniness, precisely what Freud (1985, 339) draws attention to in his essay "The Uncanny" (1919), when he makes clear the connection between *uncanny* and *unhomely*. Svenaeus (2013, 83) considers a sense of everyday embodied being which "is not a state of alienation but a state of inconspicuousness." Illness and pain disrupt this preconscious field of attention, bringing about an unhomelike being-in-the-world. It is the role of healthcare professionals to attempt to understand this "unhomelike being-in-the-world and bring it back to homelikeness again, or at least closer to a home-being" (83). He points out that bodily changes during puberty can be the source of uncanny experiences, when the body "takes on a strange life of its own that (initially at least) might feel very foreign and disgusting to the person whose body is changing" (86).

Svenaeus also discusses a case study in which the family of an adolescent girl sees the bodily alienation of anorexia as a kind of demonic possession. This leads to the suggestion that uncanniness "might foster a kind of personalization of the illness in which the anorexia is perceived as a creature with its own voice (by the anorexic girl)" (2013, 88). For Katie, as revealed in graphic representation, the personalization of illness is the black cloud, a scrawled mass of lines that acts as a visual manifestation of suffering and illness. It makes anorexia into something like a demon, which Svenaeus argues "may actually be used in attempts to help the anorexic to come to terms with her illness by externalizing it and make her see that the uncanny will and voice of her own body is actually not a necessary part of her true self" (89). Drew Leder addresses Svenaeus's description of being unable to give up anorexia. It becomes an identity, offering security and control, despite being the cause of so much suffering. It is a double experience, a perspective that "highlights the dialectical nature of a disease characterized by doubling, contradiction and paradox" (Leder 2013, 93). The anorexic, he argues, seeks transcendence through power over the body, but is trapped by the sense of being an object, overwhelmed when looking in the mirror "by the 'fat' body she is/has" (95).

Illness in *Lighter Than My Shadow* is depicted as taking hold during puberty, which for Leder (2013, 95) is a liminal phase, during which change is accompanied by a sense of discomfort: "The anorexic may wish to stop or turn back the clock, cling to the preadolescent past. However, this leads to a preoccupation with futurity. . . . Clinging to the past, focused on accomplishing future goals, the present is constricted—for example, a meal eaten slowly, one bite at a time, each calorie meticulously counted." The depiction of menstruation as a disruption of childhood, and scenes that show Katie counting and measuring her consumption of food, confirm the presence of this doubling in *Lighter Than My Shadow*. The doubling is both a seeking not to be fat and a refusing to cross the threshold of puberty (Green 2013, 44–45). This doubling reflects cultural pressures, such as the double bind of a valorization of pleasure together with moralistic judgments concerning sexuality. These are double messages: conflicted wishes lived out by the body of the anorexic. There can be a "certain self-gratifying pleasure and power" (Leder 2013, 96) together with the punishment of self-denial.

Janet Wolff (1990, 122) has argued that the body can be read as "privileged site of political intervention, precisely because it is the site of repression and possession. The body has been systematically repressed and marginal-ized in Western culture, with specific practices, ideologies, and discourses controlling and defining the female body." We see Katie monitoring herself, which is then reflexively monitored through the controlled space of critical representation. Monitoring occurs once Megan offers to give Katie a make-over in Megan's mother's room, using her makeup and dressing table mirror (Green 2013, 41). On the next page, a small panel echoes this scene, when Katie looks at her disheveled self in the mirror on the first day of secondary school (42). Later, as a dance class observe themselves in the mirrored wall of a studio, Katie self-consciously notes, "I was becoming more aware of my body" (56). This is not altogether negative, but we are shown a moment of transition, playing on doubling and the tensions between childhood and adult sexuality as discussed by Leder and Svenaeus. Katie has internalized the process of monitoring herself, and the distortions she is confronted by are defined by her expectations of conformity.

Witnessing and Graphic Form

Agamben looks at narratives of the Holocaust, at the testimonies of survi-vors, who carry the burden of bearing witness. This is not an empowered position, but one beset by guilt and shame at the very act of surviving when so many died. The position of the survivor is rendered impotent by the inability to find any justice. This shame then goes on to form a common subjectivity for all, a baseline on which postwar Western culture builds its subjects. This is an inherently problematic structure. Rather than try to identify some kind of ethics in the testimonies of survivors, which are ren-dered ineffective by shame and guilt, it is to language that we must look. In particular, it is to the breakdown of language, rather than any glimpse of meaning, which might make sense of things. Meaning can be found in the undermining of verification or certainty. The unreliability of the witness seems to suggest a questioning of our own relative stability of subjectivity, which facilitates the emergence of action, agency, and the remaking of social relations. For Agamben, the significant question is how the subject can give an account of its own ruin and destruction. *Lighter Than My Shadow* can be read as an account of the subject's ruin and destruction, but one that is able to become an act of witnessing through recovery. Redemption is part of a process of narrative visualization.

The book fits within the category of comics work that Ian Williams (2011) identifies with the process of healing in his article "Autography as Auto-Therapy: Psychic Pain the Graphic Memoir." Williams reads Justin Green's *Binky Brown Meets the Holy Virgin Mary* as a formative moment for developing a connection between autobiographical comics and healing, noting that "in 1972, [Green] became the first neurotic visionary to unburden his uncensored psychological troubles" (353). This forty-four-page comic makes use of Green's alter ego Binky Brown, who is shown trapped by an elaborate system of behavior-defining beliefs. When making the comic in the early 1970s, Green interpreted his strict upbringing among an observant Catholic family as shaping the development of his childhood compulsive neurosis. A fuller understanding of his illness came to him later: "Green was only diagnosed with Obsessive Compulsive Disorder (OCD) some time after the comic was published. At the time of his making the work the condition was ill-understood and there was no ready treatment" (Williams 2011, 354). In contrast, we see illness encroaching into all aspects of Katie's life, slowly, given form as a black cloud. Katie's family life is presented as punctuated by rituals, by a need for order and control, by a longing to be creative, specifically to draw. OCD is present and even openly addressed in Katie's childhood by her supportive and loving parents.

Illness, as a process, is intersected and addressed by another process in *Lighter Than My Shadow*—witnessing. Witnessing is a tool for aiding a recovery process, and it is due to this act of witnessing that I would like to consider the work as a zombie narrative. Williams (2012) describes a particular trait of comics, the creation of an empathic bond: "For the reader, graphic fiction can function as a portal into the individual experience of illness, laid out in the unique combination of words and text. There is so much non-propositional information packed into a comic, that the medium lends itself to very powerful narrative, creating empathic bonds between the author and the reader." In making comics, artists use a range of visual devices "to articulate the feelings associated with the illness, offering a window into the subjective realities of the author and providing companionship through shared experience in a more immediate manner."

According to Gillian Whitlock (2006, 965), the spaces between authors and readers of comics are politicized. She asks how comics can play a role in the interpretation of visual images and "their power to relay affect and invoke a moral and ethical responsiveness in the viewer regarding the suffering of others." At stake here is the question of how readers can do more than take in images of the suffering of others as passive consumers: "How can we move on to recognize the norms that govern which lives will be regarded as human, and the frames through which discourse and visual representation proceed?" (965). Whitlock coins the terms "autographics" for a conjunction of "visual and verbal text" (966). The specificity of the medium is addressed through her application of McCloud's (1994) notion of closure, as "the specific demands comics makes on the reader to produce 'closure'— the work of observing the parts but perceiving the whole" (Whitlock 2006, 969) by connecting individual panels to create a continuous and unified reality. She argues that engaging with suffering in autographics facilitates a shift in the reader, a sense of change that allows for new ways of seeing and thinking. Specifically, it is the space of the gutters between panels that creates this effect and allows for the occurrence of this form of active meaning: "This is a meaning produced in an active process of imaginative production whereby the reader shuttles between words and images, and navigates across gutters and frames, being moved to see, feel, or think differently in the effort of producing narrative closure" (978). Whitlock's reading of comics also functions in relation to Anita Helle's (2011, 298) more general account of images and narration in intersections with medicine. Writing in relation to photography, Helle looks to images as mobilizing gaps and expectations, facilitating close readings and empathic understanding, arguing that through attention to images comes agency. Images allow for the emergence of knowing, desiring, and telling selves: "They erupt at times with the velocity of sudden insight ('Aha! I see the connection now!'); at other moments, these powers emerge gradually, with the recognition that flights of thought benefit from the concretization and focus that visual artifacts and images provide" (298). For Whitlock (2006, 978), specific performing of acts of closure through the labor of reading across the gutters creates an opening through which autographics shape affective engagements.

If Whitlock focuses on the possibilities of agency afforded to the reader, Michael L. Kersulov (2014) approaches autographics as spaces for the creator to "be in control of presenting difficult memories, to explore her thoughts and reactions to traumatic moments within a safe medium, and ultimately to construct herself on the page." This can be a making sense of events in the past, giving meaning not only to memories but also to the person the author has decided to be in the present. There is an empowering of authors through how they depict and re-create situations in which they did not have control: "Choosing how they depict the scene, characters, action, dialogue, etc. mimics not only how they remember the event but also how they choose to counteract it." Acts of witnessing are addressed in more specific detail by Emily Waples (2014, 156) and her application of the term autopathographics (comics as personal narratives relating to illness or disability) that contest stigmatization and pathological discourses that cast the author as abnormal: "Inviting audiences into the intimate spaces of illness, autopathogragraphic narratives implicate the reader as a witness to the often uncomfortable vicissitudes of embodied experience." Waples builds on ideas of performing illness through graphic media, calling attention to the boundaries of representation. She studies representations of breast cancer as resistant to narrative closure due to "its possibility of metastasizing many years after its diagnosis" (158) and explores the possibilities of graphic forms to "register the uncertainty of the disease's temporality" (159). Autopathographics highlight what is seen and not seen, illuminating relationships to the disciplinary frameworks of medical discourse.

Sarah Lightman discusses "imagiastic possession" in the telling of harrowing stories, taking Cathy Caruth's statement that "to be traumatized is precisely to be possessed of an image" (Caruth 1995, cited in Lightman 2014, 201). Lightman deviates from Caruth's take on trauma as an involuntary revisiting by selecting three voluntary returns to the scenes of traumatic events in three autobiographical graphic novels. Katie Green's book fits alongside Lightman's selection of Sarah Leavitt's *Tangles: A Story about Alzheimer's, My Mother, and Me* (2011), Nicola Streeten's *Billy, Me, and You: A Memoir of Grief and Recovery* (2011), and Maureen Burdock's *Mona and the Little Smile* (2008). Lightman identifies common elements between these three works, which they share with Green's book. To start, they were all written a number of years after the events depicted. "Secondly," Lightman (2014, 202) writes, "all three women are self-taught comic artists and their books were either their first published graphic novels, or in Burdock's case, her first series of published comics. Thirdly, the publication of these books has had a positive and transformational effect on the life of the authors and others." Lightman suggests that personal and professional growth can be achieved as a transformational result of trauma and tragedy, and reads this trajectory into a number of theories of narratives of illness, citing Arthur Frank's *The Wounded Storyteller* among others. Frank "discusses how creating a narrative of illness and recovery helps patients to gain control of their experiences" (Lightman 2014, 202). The roots of the comics Lightman discusses are *herstories*, women narrating their own lives. Lightman holds up Diane Noomin and Aline Kominsky-Crumb as formative examples: "These life stories happened in internalized spaces: miscarriages inside the woman's body, sexual and spouse abuse within the family, in the family home. Comics, in their constructed and contained world of panels and borders, offer a space both closed and open to the public. These everyday stories that previously had been silenced, or kept hidden in cultures of silence, find a voice and a space on the comics' page" (202). Of Leavitt, Streeton, and Burdock, Lightman argues that in "creative responses they have found healing, communities, and perhaps most importantly audiences who can validate and appreciate their experiences. By taking traumatic experiences and making them visible and visual, these three women have found a posttraumatic life of positive possibilities" (215).

This sense of practical possibility does not relate to therapy. Therapy is represented early on in *Lighter Than My Shadow*. We are shown a family therapy session, taking place in the early stages of the eating disorder, with Katie and her younger sister laughing together about how Katie had hidden her toast instead of eating it (Green 2013, 21). On the following page a contrasting process is represented. Whereas therapy is shown as, at the very least, an inefficient and not wholly adequate approach to creating well-being and stable subject formation, drawing as narrative is presented as a hopeful promise in the midst of an increasing sense of illness. A caption accompanying images of young Katie drawing reads, "There was always something better to do than eating," but it also suggests that there was something better than talking: "I was happiest playing alone . . . living in my imagination . . . and I preferred not to be interrupted" (22). A splash page leads us from Katie leaning over a table, drawing, into a world of fantasy, which then transitions into a sheet of paper before Katie as she lies on the floor but is interrupted by her mother's call. This is echoed two pages later as we see Katie reading in bed; the content of her book is the destination of a flow of water, complete with fish, running down from an idealized landscape that hovers across the top of the page (24). Katie is shown finding happiness between the space of reading and narrative drawing as a practice. The next page completes the assembly of these elements. In the first panel Katie's mother asks what she is drawing, to which Katie responds:

"It's a story . . ."
"Your own story?"
"Yup." (25)

There is a play on drawing your own story. Of course the mother means a story of Katie's own invention, but the resonance is that this girl is drawing her own story, as in *herstory*. In the final panel on the page we see Katie at the front of the class at school in a show-and-tell session, presenting her childish drawings to the class, saying, "When I grow up, I'm going to do picture books like this . . ." (25). This is a promise that we know will be ultimately fulfilled, and it cannot be detached from the process of recovery and the act of witnessing enabled by the book. However, these hopeful and optimistic elements are immediately undermined by darker fantasy imagery, a realm of fear that can only be countered by the introduction of rituals. Food is included in this ritualized approach, a clear and explanatory link between different behaviors.

Rituals and control develop within the happy and stable home environment. While a balance can be maintained, so can a sense of normalcy. However, a happy scene of Katie helping her mother make a cake leads to some poignant questioning:

> "What happens if you don't eat?" asks Katie.
> "Well, you'd just fade away . . . into oblivion," her mother replies.
> "What's a blivion?" (33)

From this point onward, we are introduced to a scrawling mass, a squiggle that forms the black cloud that follows and hovers above Katie. A set of panels depicts Katie's body reducing over time, as the cloud increases. A caption reads, "Years later, I learned what oblivion meant" (34).

A jump in the narrative on the opposite page depicts an older Katie as the teller of this story. She sits at a desk grasping a pen, with a mug, notes, and a drawing of the black scribble cloud. She is crying (35).

She sits at the bottom of the page and a vast black cloud wisps above her, as if a monstrous speech bubble. We see that she has not faded into oblivion, but that the manifestation of that fear or desire still haunts her, that this is an active and ongoing process. The narrating Katie Green asks, "Were these early signs of an eating disorder?" (36). She also comments that her only memories were of being happy. However, this changes as Katie enters secondary school. One particular ongoing situation leads to the taunts of a group of boys becoming a cursive, semi-legible scrawl that follows her like the black cloud. When she gets home, rather than tell her parents about the incident she forages for snack food and takes it to her room. As she begins to eat, the words collapse in a three-panel sequence until they are just visible at the bottom of the third panel as a haunting, scribbly black shadow (53). Shame and embarrassment, social encounters around food, and her growing sense of self-doubt are increasingly accompanied by the black cloud.

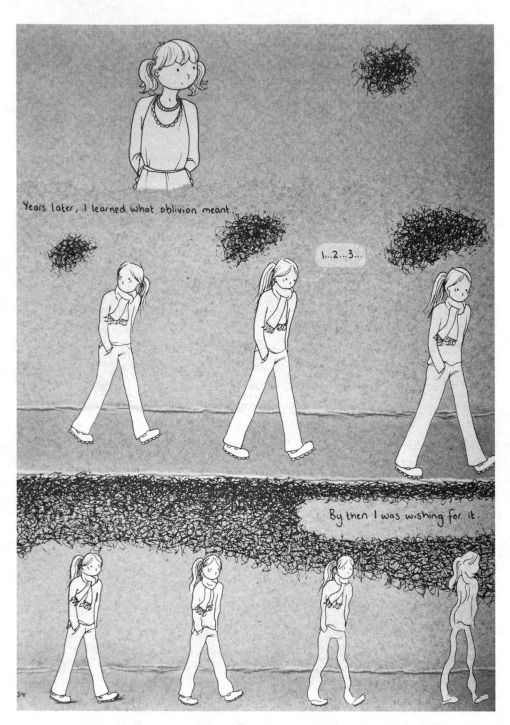

9.4 From *Lighter Than My Shadow* by Katie Green, published by Jonathan Cape. Reproduced by permission of The Random House Group Ltd.

The cloud can be held at bay through academic endeavor, by immersing herself in homework. However, academic success leads to further social alienation and becomes an excuse for avoiding social contact with her peers. Another layer of alienation is depicted in the frustrating of her own creative ambitions at school, which might be interpreted here as an inability to act as a witnessing subject. A specific example is Katie's fear of the blank page, which makes her hesitate and fail to demonstrate creativity in art classes. Despite stating that she would like to be an illustrator, her careers adviser explains that she is not suitable for this career. She is told to concentrate on other subjects such as mathematics, sciences, and languages. This interruption accelerates her decline, closing off a space for exploring and establishing her own subjectivity, propelling her toward the conditions of becoming zombielike.

9.5 From *Lighter Than My Shadow* by Katie Green, published by Jonathan Cape. Reproduced by permission of The Random House Group Ltd.

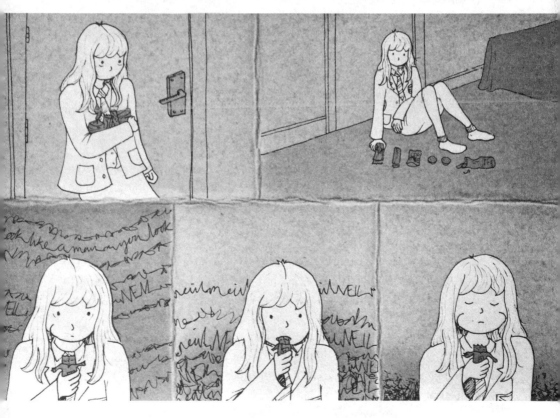

In a three-panel sequence we are shown Katie in a dream, her naked body surrounded by the cloud and expanding, as if swelling with pregnancy. Katie maps out her thigh and stomach with dotted lines that, as Kevin Ezra Moore (2014, 228) discusses, denote both surgery and butchery. The final panel shows Katie slicing away part of her thigh with a cleaver. This is a horrific moment visualizing her making her body inhuman and not living: an image of herself as already dead, an unfeeling thing that can be cut to pieces, reshaped as a piece of meat (Green 2013, 101).

The vividness of this internal position is shown clearly to readers, as is the futility of Katie's attempt to explain her feelings to her mother, who simply assures her that she is not fat, that she has a "lovely figure" (103). This is the repeated gap between what her own family cannot see and what Green can show us in the graphic form. Another such gap is present in an apparently innocent scene where the family and the dog are sitting in their living room sharing a box of chocolates (104–5). As Katie eats one, gently pressured by her mother, we see the black cloud start to form in Katie's throat as she begins to swallow, traveling down and expanding into her body. This is food as foreign, as alien (Svenaeus 2013, 87). As Katie gets up and walks away from her family, the cloud also forms in the space between her and her family, forming a barrier visible to us but not to them. Green is able to exploit the medium in which she works to generate her specific manifestations of body horror.

Surviving the Zombie, Becoming Human

Lighter Than My Shadow is a representation of illness that explores biological and social boundaries of living. As closer to death than life, as an embodied subject who has almost become a walking cadaver, Katie goes through a process of dehumanization and alienation. Yet this is a zombie narrative that ultimately depicts and facilitates a process of remaking the subject. Self-reflection and representation become part of a process of active engagement and re-empowerment, of becoming human. Katie is shown approaching a threshold, that of the Muselmann as a kind of zombie, yet she is also shown returning from this impossible threshold. *Lighter Than My Shadow* is consistent with zombie narratives that seek agency for the zombie, the possibility of life after becoming a zombie. The unconditional fatalism of the Muselmann is overcome, as is the colonization of illness and health by industrial systems.

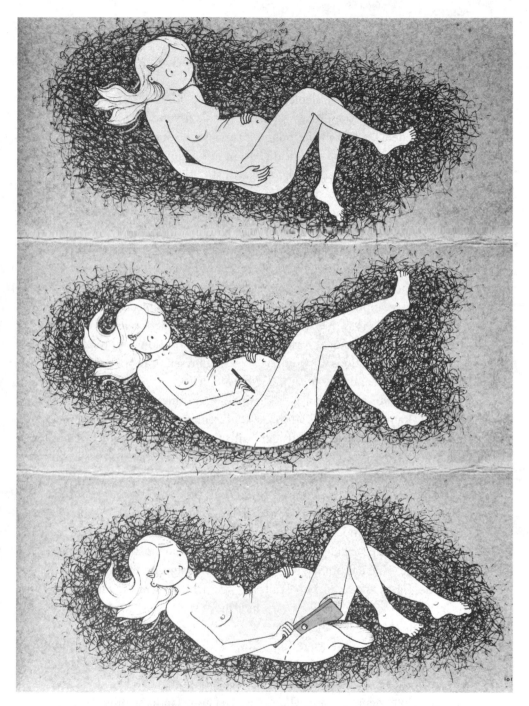

9.6 From *Lighter Than My Shadow* by Katie Green, published by Jonathan Cape. Reproduced by permission of The Random House Group Ltd.

The process of healing has not been brought about through the book as such, but was necessary before the book could be made. Creating *Lighter Than My Shadow* was a part of a larger process, including both successes and failures. There are depictions of counseling in the book, but counseling did not prevent the events depicted from taking place or forestall the need for the book itself. The process of creating this five-hundred-page work cannot be detached from the ongoing process of Green's recovery, and should be recognized as a significant part of this ongoing process. The level of attentive detail required, of planning, constructing, of consistent execution of images and character design across so much space, for example, demands a redirecting of the otherwise potentially destructive obsessive tendencies depicted in the narrative. The process of making the work, as well as its thematic and narrative content, are characterized by the application of such tendencies as part of a coming to terms with patterns of behavior and thinking that cannot be expelled entirely, but might be controlled. The creation of the book is an act of reforming subjectivity, echoing Catherine Itzin's (1987, 116) demand for writing to function as an actively oppositional performance working against the institutional reproduction of oppressive conditions for women: "Creating myself is a continuing process of discharge and re-evaluation."

Lighter Than My Shadow is not reducible to some form of therapy or catharsis. Rather, the book is a form of representation and re-presentation, in which we see Katie Green struggle with the image of herself as well as construct a space of agency and understanding. The zombie emerges as an extreme manifestation in this struggle for agency. The almost-unliving body is at the center of an act of witnessing that must be made difficult, a process of understanding that must acknowledge that there are no simple explanations. As Lesley Saunders (1987, 160) points out, for women, writing themselves on the page is rehabilitation, due to an impression instilled in women as being the Other, as not having a fully realized subjectivity. As a process, this is described as painful, but "exhilarating in achievement." The transition from Katie's most zombielike states to a more stable human subjectivity reflects this process of realization.

Her return from the condition of a withered collection of barely functioning body parts is prefigured by appearances in the work of an adult Katie but is also charted within the narrative. Visually, motifs of a new dress and haircut help to depict a Katie who has moved away from the inhuman, unalive state of her most ill self.

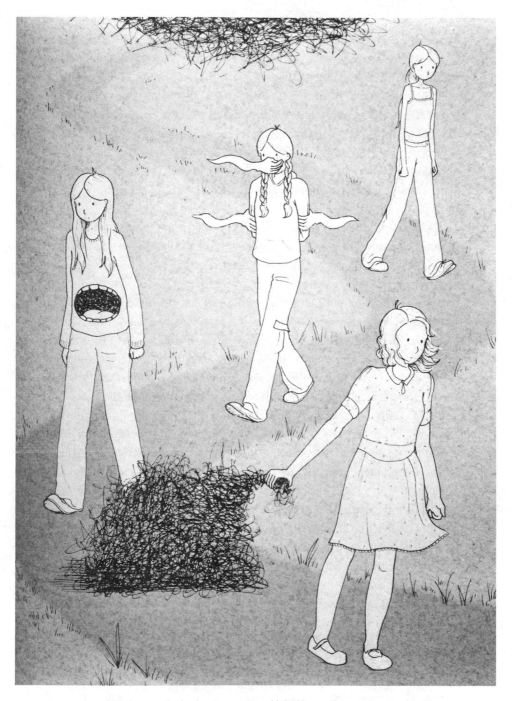

9.7 From *Lighter Than My Shadow* by Katie Green, published by Jonathan Cape. Reproduced by permission of The Random House Group Ltd.

These two superficial elements should not be conflated with elements of normative gender performativity—those are the conditions that facilitated illness in the first place—but rather serve to generate visualized differences in the transition between younger Katie and her contemporary, healthier self. This transitional Katie is still subject to binges and insecurity but is able to listen to reassuring voices within herself (Green 2013, 482). This is a marked transition from bodily emaciation and the loss of agency that creates the zombielike Katie. As a zombie, Katie's subjectivity disintegrates. We see her reintegrated, through Katie Green's drawings and through images of Katie drawing, a performing and reiteration of subjective reintegration through drawing.

As a zombie narrative, *Lighter Than My Shadow* offers sympathetic understandings of the existential challenges that can lead to illness and suggests paths to recovery. Image/text combinations, the juxtaposition of images, and the control of temporality in narrative form all add to this layered encounter that facilitates empathy, engagement, and understanding. The flexibility that the medium of comics possesses in processing time—which I have described in detail elsewhere (Smith 2013)—is put to use to reconfigure the body as a process rather than a thing, by revealing change visually, temporally, and psychically. The body is also configured as something existing between anatomical fact and a realm of emotional experience and metaphor. The cold clarity of the body as Muselmann is unflinchingly depicted across the pages of *Lighter Than My Shadow*, a fact of physical emaciation that Katie was at the time unable to recognize. For Green to show herself is to reveal what the character could not see. This act of witnessing and representation is not a healing process in itself but becomes a way to build on healing, another step in the ongoing process of dealing with her illness. Katie moves from a withered collection of neurotically driven bodily functions to a subject able to trouble the normative frameworks that made her condition possible. To approach becoming a Muselmann, to become zombie, and yet to return from it, suggests a challenge to the normative conditions that enabled the illness to take hold of Katie. By indirectly evoking a precursor of the zombie, Green provides a figure that questions boundaries of life and death.

REFERENCES

Agamben, Giorgio. 2002. *Remnants of Auschwitz: The Witness and the Archive.* Translated by Daniel Heller-Roazen. New York: Zone Books.

Bishop, Kyle William. 2010. *American Zombie Gothic: The Rise and Fall (and Rise) of the Walking Dead in Popular Culture.* Jefferson, NC: McFarland.

————. 2015. "I've Always Wanted to See How the Other Half Lives: The Contemporary Zombie as Seductive Proselyte." In *The Zombie Renaissance in Popular Culture*, edited by Laura Hubner, Marcus Leaning, and Paul Manning, 26–40. London: Palgrave Macmillan.

Blanchot, Maurice. 1995. *The Writing of the Disaster*. Translated by Ann Smock. Lincoln: University of Nebraska Press.

Caruth, Cathy. 1995. Introduction. In *Trauma: Explorations in Memory*, edited by Cathy Caruth, 3–12. Baltimore: Johns Hopkins University Press.

Cazdyn, Eric. 2012. *The Already Dead: The New Time of Politics, Culture, and Illness*. Durham, NC: Duke University Press.

Clasen, Mathias. 2010. "The Anatomy of the Zombie: A Bio-Psychological Look at the Undead Other." *Otherness: Essays and Studies* 1 (1): 1–23.

El Refaie, Elisabeth. 2012. *Autobiographical Comics: Life Writing in Pictures*. Jackson: University Press of Mississippi.

Freud, Sigmund. 1985. "The Uncanny." In *Penguin Freud 14: Art and Literature*, edited by Albert Dickson, 335–76. London: Penguin.

Green, Katie. 2013. *Lighter Than My Shadow*. London: Jonathan Cape.

————. 2014. "Lighter Than My Shadow." http://katiegreen.co.uk/books/lighter -than-my-shadow/.

Helle, Anita. 2011. "When the Photograph Speaks: Photo-Analysis in Narrative Medicine." *Literature and Medicine* 29 (2): 297–324.

Itzin, Catharine. 1987. "Head, Hand, Heart— and the Writing of Wrongs." In *Glancing Fires: An Investigation into Women's Creativity*, edited by Lesley Saunders, 115–20. London: Women's Press.

Kersulov, Michael L. 2014. "Making Serious Subjects Lighter: Trauma in the Adolescent Autographic." *ImageTexT* 7 (4). http://www.english.ufl.edu/imagetext/ archives/v7_4/kersulov/.

Leder, Drew. 2013. "Anorexia: A Disease of Doubling." *Philosophy, Psychiatry, and Psychology* 20 (1): 93–96.

Lightman, Sarah. 2014. "Metamorphosing Difficulties: The Portrayal of Trauma in Autobiographical Comics." In *The Unspeakable: Narratives of Trauma*, edited by Magda Stroinska, Vikki Cecchetto, and Kate Szymanski, 201–27. Frankfurt: Peter Lang.

McCloud, Scott. 1994. *Understanding Comics: The Invisible Art*. New York: Harper Perennial.

Moore, Kevin Ezra. 2014. *The Spatial Language of Time: Metaphor, Metonymy, and Frames of Reference*. Amsterdam: John Benjamins.

Platts, Todd. 2013. "Locating Zombies in the Sociology of Popular Culture." *Sociology Compass* 7 (7): 547–60.

Saunders, Lesley. 1987. "Hollering from the Earth: Form." In *Glancing Fires: An Investigation into Women's Creativity*, edited by Lesley Saunders, 159–60. London: Women's Press.

Smith, Dan. 2013. "Architecture, Violence, and Sensation: A Visitor's Guide to Mega-City One." *Intensities: The Journal of Cult Media* 5 (Spring –Summer). http://intensitiescult media.com/issue-5-springsummer -2013/.

Sontag, Susan. 1991. *"Illness as Metaphor" and "AIDS and Its Metaphors."* London: Penguin.

Svenaeus, Fredrik. 2013. "Anorexia Nervosa and the Body Uncanny: A Phenomenological Approach." *Philosophy, Psychiatry, and Psychology* 20 (1): 81–104.

Waples, Emily. 2014. "Avatars, Illness, and Authority: Embodied Experience in Breast Cancer Autopathographics." *Configurations* 22 (2): 153–81.

Whitlock, Gillian. 2006. "Autographics: The Seeing I of the Comics." *Modern Fiction Studies* 52 (4): 965–79.

Williams, Ian. 2011. "Autography as Auto- Therapy: Psychic Pain and the Graphic

Memoir." *Journal of Medical Humanities* 32 (4): 353–66.
———. 2012. "Graphic Medicine." *Hektoen
International: A Journal of Medical
Humanities* 4 (1). http://www.hektoen

international.org/index.php?option
=com_content&view=article&id=353.
Wolff, Janet. 1990. *Feminine Sentences: Essays
on Women and Culture*. Malden, MA:
Polity Press.

CON-
TRIBU-
TORS

Tully Barnett is a Research Fellow in the School of Humanities and Creative Arts, Flinders University in South Australia, where she works on a project investigating cultural value in the creative arts. She also publishes on technologies of reading such as Kindle social highlighting and Google Books marginalia. Her PhD thesis examined representations of information technology in contemporary literary fiction. She is the author of "Monstrous Agents: Cyberfeminist Digital Media and Activism," published by *Ada: A Journal of Gender, New Media, and Technology* in 2014; "'Reading Saved Me': Transformative Reading Experiences in Life Narrative," by *Prose Studies: History, Theory, Criticism* in 2013; "Repackaging Popular Culture: Commentary and Critique in Community" (co-authored with Ben Kooyman), by *Networking Knowledge* in 2012; and "Remediating the Infected Body: Writing the Viral Self in Melinda Rackham's Carrier," by *Biography* in 2012.

Gerry Canavan is an Assistant Professor in the English Department at Marquette University, teaching twentieth- and twenty-first-century literature. His current research projects include *Science Fiction and Totality* and *Modern Masters of Science Fiction: Octavia E. Butler*, as well as co-editing *The Cambridge Companion to American Science Fiction* and *Green Planets: Ecology and Science Fiction*.

Daniel George is a member of the Department of Humanities at Penn State College of Medicine. He earned his BA from the College of Wooster and his PhD and MSc in medical anthropology from Oxford University. George is co-author of *The Myth of Alzheimer's: What You Aren't Being Told about Today's Most Dreaded Diagnosis*, published by St. Martin's Press in 2008. In addition to teaching and research at Penn State, George serves as the director of the farmers market in Hershey and has helped establish a community garden on the hospital campus. In his spare time he enjoys painting, playing guitar in a Beatles cover band, and gritting through *The Walking Dead* television series.

Michael Green is a Professor of Medicine and Humanities at Penn State College of Medicine, where he cares for patients, teaches medical students, and conducts research on informed medical decision making. He is a founding organizer of several international conferences on comics and medicine and a member of the editorial collective of a book series on graphic medicine from Penn State University Press. He teaches a course called "Comics and Medicine" to fourth-year medical students, whose comics can be viewed online at http://www2.med.psu.edu/. He has published the first comic to appear in the *Annals of Internal Medicine* and academic articles on comics and medicine in *BMJ* and the *Journal of Medical Humanities*. Green also has numerous publications on medical education and bioethics.

Ben Kooyman graduated from Flinders University in 2010 with a PhD in English. His dissertation dealt with Shakespeare, film, and self-fashioning. He currently works as a language and learning adviser at the University of South Australia. His research interests include horror cinema, Australian film, Shakespeare, comic books, and adaptation studies. His first book, titled *Directorial Self-Fashioning in American Horror Cinema: George A. Romero, Wes Craven, Rob Zombie, Eli Roth, and the Masters of Horror*, was published by Edwin Mellen in 2014.

Sarah Juliet Lauro is the co-author of "A Zombie Manifesto: The Nonhuman Condition in the Era of Advanced Capitalism," published by *boundary 2* in 2008, and co-editor of *Better Off Dead: The Evolution of the Zombie as Posthuman*, published by Fordham University Press in 2011. Her first book, *The Transatlantic Zombie: Slavery, Rebellion, and Living Death*, was published by Rutgers University Press in 2015. She is an Assistant Professor of English at the University of Tampa.

Juliet McMullin, PhD, specializes in cultural and medical anthropology at the University of California, Riverside. She has recently been appointed Director of Healthy Communities at the UC Riverside Medical School. She is the author of *The Healthy Ancestor: Embodied Inequality and the Revital-*

ization of Native Hawaiian Health and co-editor of the School of Advanced Research volume *Confronting Cancer: Metaphors, Advocacy, and Anthropology*. Professor McMullin has had an enduring interest in the production of health knowledge and inequalities. Her research, far from naturalizing health as solely a biological process, examines the contexts in which political struggles over health embody inequality and reflect efforts at reconfiguring individual subjectivities and social structures. She is the lead organizer for the Center for Ideas and Society Medical Narratives workgroup and was recently awarded a National Endowment for the Humanities Humanities Initiatives grant on medical narratives. Her current research is situated in the field of graphic medicine. This work is both an examination of the social and material role of graphic novels in narrative medicine and health inequalities, and an ethnography of community building.

Kari Nixon is a postdoctoral fellow at Southern Methodist University, where her research focuses on contagious disease in literature—particularly that of the fin de siècle. Her essay on hemorrhaging sores in Daniel Defoe's *A Journal of the Plague Year* is forthcoming in the *Journal for Early Modern Cultural Studies*, and her essay on the cultural contexts of *Jane Eyre* is forthcoming in the second edition of *Jane Eyre* in the Bedford / St. Martin's critical casebook series. She has presented at multiple international conferences on the topic of contagious disease in literature, including MLA, SLSA, and NAVSA. She has recently been named graduate liaison to the executive committee of SLSA and elected a graduate representative of NAVSA. She has recently been awarded funding from the King Olav V Norwegian-American Heritage Fund to conduct archival research in Oslo and is currently in residence as a guest researcher at the Centre for Ibsen Studies, conducting research on Ibsen and syphilis.

Steve Schlozman is an Assistant Professor of Psychiatry and Co-Director of Medical Student Education in Psychiatry at Harvard Medical School. He has published over thirty articles on psychiatry and medical education and is the author of *The Zombie Autopsies* (a novel), which is currently being adapted into a film with George Romero. Schlozman has published numerous subsequent periodicals and editorials on zombies in venues such as the *New York Times*. He has also given a number of talks on zombies vis-à-vis neuroscience, including one at the King's College Narrative Medicine Conference in 2013.

Lorenzo Servitje is a PhD candidate in English at the University of California, Riverside. His research focuses on the intersection of Victorian literature and medical history. His articles and reviews have appeared in *Journal of Medical Humanities*, *Critical Survey*, and *Science Fiction Studies*, and two articles are forthcoming in *Literature and Medicine*. He is also co-editor of *Endemic: Essay in Contagion Theory*, to be published by Palgrave in 2016.

Dan Smith is a Senior Lecturer in Fine Art Theory in the BA Fine Art course at Chelsea College of Arts, London. He is the author of *Traces of Modernity* and *Agamben Reframed*. Current areas of interest include science fiction, utopia, comics, museology, and material culture. Recent publications include "Reading Folk Archive: On the Utopian Dimension of the Artists' Book" in *Literatures, Libraries, and Archives*, and "Image, Technology, and Enchantment: Interview with Marina Warner" in *The Machine and the Ghost: Technology and Spiritualism in Nineteenth- to Twenty-First-Century Art and Culture*. His drawings can be found at http://danthatdraws.blogspot.com/.

Sherryl Vint is Professor of English and Director of the Speculative Fiction and Cultures of Science program at the University of California, Riverside. An editor of the journals *Science Fiction Film and Television* and *Science Fiction Studies*, she has published widely on speculative fiction.

Darryl Wilkinson is an Andrew W. Mellon postdoctoral fellow in the Center for the Humanities at the University of Wisconsin-Madison. He received his training in anthropology from Columbia University and Oxford University and currently conducts fieldwork in two locations: the cloud forests of southern Peru and the Rio Grande region of northern New Mexico. His research examines the ways indigenous forms of religion are expressed through material and visual culture, as well as how they have changed over time, from prehistory up until the colonial era.

INDEX

Page numbers in *italics* refer to illustrations.

antibiotics, 41, 61
antisocial behaviors, 81, 84, 86. *See also* cannibalism; violence
anxiety, 22
aphasia, 18, 24
appetite, 29–30, 34, 57, 60, 62–63. *See also* anorexia; consumption
Aquilina, Carmelo, 21, 36
Aragon, Alejandro, 124
Archer, James, 140n2. See also *Preparedness 101: Zombie Pandemic* (Silver, et al.)
Archie Comics, 37n9
Ariès, Philippe, 148
Ashcroft, Bill, 68
As I Lay Dying (Faulkner), 147
Ataxic Neurodegenerative Satiety Syndrome (ANSD), 171, 173–78, *176,* 179–83, *181*
Atwood, Margaret, 26
Auschwitz concentration camp, 192, 194, 195, 197–98
autism, 50
autobiographical comics, 200, 203. See also *Lighter Than My Shadow* (Green, K.)
Autobiographical Comics (El Refaie), 200
autographics, 204–5
"Autography as Auto-Therapy" (Williams), 203
autopathographics, 205
autopsies, 175–83, *180, 181. See also* dissection
avian flu, 3, 124
Away from Her (Polley film), 21

Baartman, Saartjie, 147
Baena, Jeff, 37n5, 55, 191
Bakhtin, Mikhail, 166–67n9
Ballard, J. G., 153–54, 160
Banbury, Trey: "Perspective," 87, *88,* 90–91, *92*
bare life, 196, 197
Barnes, Djuna, 146–47, 149
Bartholomew, Saint, 157, 160
Bashford, Alison, 58
bath salts, 3
Bath Salt Zombies (film), 10n2
Becerra, Gaspar: flayed cadaver etchings, 153, *154,* 157
Becoming Biosubjects (Gerlach, Hamilton, Sullivan, and Walton), 139
behavior alterations, 4, 18, 20, 26, 27, 29, 174
Behuniak, Susan M., 21, 27, 76
Being and Time (Heidegger), 148–49

"Being a Patient Made Me a More Empathic (Future) Doctor" (Holmes), 93–94, *94*
Beisecker, Dave, 24, 53n3
Bell, John, 167n10
Benjamin, Walter, 185, 187n14
Bichat, Xavier, 171, 172, 178
Bicycle Girl (*Walking Dead* character), 44, *45*
Bidloo, Govard: *Ontleding des menschelyken lichaams,* 153, *155,* 156
Big Daddy (*Land of the Dead* character), 157
Billy, Me, and You (Streeten), 205
Binky Brown Meets the Holy Virgin Mary (Green, J.), 203
bioethics, 172, 175–78
biopolitics, 13, 66, 91, 156, 202–4. *See* Agamben, Foucault, and Mbembe
bioterrorism, 136, 137, 139
Birth of the Clinic, The (Foucault), 171–72
birth rate statistics, 19
Bishop, Kyle, 82, 191
Blackest Night (DC Comics), 27–28, 29
Blackest Night: The Flash (Johns and Reis), 28
Blackgas (Ellis, Fiumara, and Waterhouse), 26, *27*
Black Lanterns, 27–28
Blanca Guiterrez (*Zombie Autopsies* character), 172
Blanchot, Maurice, 192, 195
blood mists (visual motif), 134
body degeneration. *See also* cognitive function
   anorexia, 191, 192, 214
   corpse decomposition, 152
   drugs causing, 3
   elderly, 18, 20–24, 26, 27–29
   Holocaust victims, 192, 194
   zombie disease progression and nonhuman classifications based on, 42, 172, 175–78, *176*
   zombie medical illustrations, 156–61, *157, 158, 159, 161*
   of zombies, 18, 24, 29, 42, 60, 61
Body Worlds (Hagens), 147, 157
Boer Wars, 69n4
Boney, Roy, Jr., 33–37, *35*
border crashers, 162
bovine spongiform encephalopathy ("Mad Cow Disease"), 174
Bowes (*New Edwardian* character), 58
Boyle, Danny. See *28 Days Later* (Boyle film)

brain cannibalism, 187n6

brain-dead humans

life support debates, 106

medico-legal constructions for death definitions, 176, 177

organ harvesting on, *96*, 96–99, *97*, *98*, 176,
177

zombification and nonhuman classifications of, 172, 175–78

brain degeneration, 26, 30, 173–78, 183, 187n6,
194

brain imaging, 175–76, *176*, 179–86, *180*

brain studies. *See* neurobiology

Bright, the (*New Deadwardians* human characters), 56, 57, 60, 64, 66

Britain, 55–60, 64–66, 138

Brooks, Max, 60

Brown, Bill, 149, 150–51

Brown, Michael, 151

Browne, John, 150

Burdine, Troy Simon, II, 147

Burdock, Maureen, 205, 206

Burke, William, 146

Burri, Regula Valérie, 8

Burrows, Jacen, *49*, *51*

Butler, Judith, 132

caffeine consumption, *82*, 83, 86

"Camp Chemo Plan, Summer 1995" from *Soldier's Heart* (Tyler), 111–12, *112*

cancer

chemicals causing, 108–9, 110, 111–13, *113*,
116–19, *117*, *118*

chemicals treating (*see* chemotherapy)

as geriatric illness, 18, 20, 22

graphic medicine and emotional experience of, 127

human body presence and agency of, 107

patients as zombie metaphors, 105, *105*,
116–17, *118*

treatment costs and patient oppression, 108

Cancer Made Me a Shallower Person (Engelberg), 105, *105*, 120

Cancer Vixen (Marchetto), 114–16, 120

cannibalism

neurodegenerative diseases caused by, 174,
187n6

as zombie characteristic, 21, 28–29, 60,
166n9, 176

capitalism, global, 76, 117, 164, 165, 196

Captain Boomerang I (*Blackest Night* character), 28

Captain Boomerang II (*Blackest Night* character), 28

Captain Cold (*Blackest Night* character), 28

Captain West (*28 Days Later* character), 140n3

Carey, M. R., 26

Carl (*Walking Dead* character), 46

Carstairs (*New Deadwardian* character), 67

Carter, Henry Vandyke, 182

Carter, Richard, 147

cartography, 66

Cartwright, Lisa, 9, 184

Caruth, Cathy, 205

"Case of the Fearless Rat, The," 7–8

Cassavetes, Nick, 21

Casserio, Giulio, 160–61, *162*

Cazdyn, Eric, 6, 10n9, 196–97

CDC (Centers for Disease Control and Pre-
vention), 3, 124, 172. *See also*
Preparedness 101: Zombie Pandemic
(Silver, et al.)

Celia (*New Deadwardian* character), 67

chemical embodiment, 107, 111–12

chemically transformed beings, 108–9, 114, 118

chemical regimes of life, 106, 111, 113–14, 116,
119–20

chemicals

bioterrorism, 136, 137, 139

cancer-causing, 108–9, 110, 111–14, *112*, *113*,
116–19, *117*, *118*, 120

cancer-treating (*see* chemotherapy)

modern global and economic pervasion of,
106, 109, 111, 113–14, 116, 119–20

chemo brain, 107, 115

chemotherapy

contradictory advice for, 114–15

cost and healthcare accessibility, 108

function, 106

historical use and origins of, 106

as life/death zombie toxin, 107, 110–12, *112*,
114

long-term consequences of, 62

side effects of, 107, 110, 114, 115

war metaphors and, 110, 111, 115–16, 120

cholera epidemics, 66

chronic disease conditions, 6, 33–34, 196–97

cigarette smoking, 116–19, *117*, *118*

civil rights issues
  nonhuman classifications and medical
    experimentation, 175, 176
  public panic consequences, 32, 33, 35, 125–
    26, 127, 139–40
Clarens, Carlos, 33
Clarke, Adele, 10n1
Clasen, Mathias, 191
Clint Harris (*28 Days Later* comic character)
  bioterrorism themes and air travel scenes,
    136
  dehumanization of sick, 137–38
  grievability themes, 132
  memorial wall visitation, 138
  normalcy of repatriation, 139
  plot and character description, 124
  wartime politics, 133–34
closure, 204
coffee consumption, *82, 83,* 86
cognitive function. *See also* brain-dead
    humans
  anorexia and self-concept distortions, 192
  caffeine requirements for, 83
  chemotherapy side effects and loss of, 107,
    115
  drugs impacting, 2–3, 4
  hunger-induced dysfunction, 28–29
  neurobiology and humanity based on, 177
  neurodegeneration, 26, 30, 173–78, 183,
    187n6, 194
  personality alterations, 4, 18, 20, 26, 27, 29,
    174
  zombies with heightened, 41, 48, 50, 52
  zombies with lack/loss of, 47, 50
Cohen, Jeffrey Jerome, 151–52
Cold War, 86, 132
colonialism, 57–59, 65, 66, 132–33, 165–66
color symbolism, 65–66, 134
"Comics and Medicine" (Penn State College of
    Medicine course), 77–79
communication, 18–19, 24–29, 32–36
Complete treatise of the muscles, A (Browne),
    160
Configurations (journal), 126–27
conformity, 86–87, 202
Conner, Mark, 140n2. See also *Preparedness
    101: Zombie Pandemic* (Silver, et al.)
Conrad, Peter, 56
consumption (consumerism)

of cancer-causing toxins, 109, 116–19, *117,*
  118
  medical student comic theme, *82, 83,*
    83–86, *84, 85*
  as zombie characteristic, 28–29, 60, 95,
    166n9, 176
  as zombie narrative theme, 76, 82–83, 123
contagion. *See* viruses and viral epidemics
Contagion (Soderbergh film), 131
*Contagious: Cultures, Carriers and the Out-
    break Narrative* (Wald), 5, 55, 58, 65,
    132–33, 137
containment
  family empathy and response, 24, 25
  for future treatment, 46–47
  geographic space and illness associations,
    57, 64–65, 66
  government policies, 131
  institutionalization, 32, 33, 35
  public panic and response, 124, 125, 126,
    129, 138, 139–40
corpses
  as abjection representations, 106, 110
  artistic zombification of, 156–61
  decay process descriptions, 152
  dementia patients as walking, 21–22
  exploitation and exhibition of, 147
  in literature, 146–47
  living as walking, 152–53
  medical illustrations of, in history, 153–54,
    160, 160–61, *162,* 167n10–11
  as medical school anatomical models, 146,
    151, 153–54, 171–72
  object-oriented ontology of, 148–51
  types and uses of, 146
  viewing experiences, 145–46
  in visual arts, 147
  zombie-oriented ontology of, 151–52, 165
"Cost Conundrum, The" (Gawande), 40
Creutzfeldt-Jakob disease, 174
Crossed (Ennis)
  digital virality and desensitization, 48, 49
  human normalcy *vs.* nonhuman altered
    state, *49,* 50
  viral infection narrative assumptions, 42
  viral infection theme and epidemic defini-
    tions, 40, 41
  zombie descriptions, 41, 48, 50, *51,* 52
Crucifixion imagery, 63

cryogenics, 6
"Crypt, The" (*Zombie Autopsies* research site), 172, 173
Culbard, I. N. J., 55, 59, 60
"Cure, The" (*New Deadwardians* medical intervention), 55, 56–57, 60–63, 67–68
cysticercosis, 10n7

Dana (*Revival* character), 30–33
Daston, Lorraine, 8–9, 170, 180–81, 182, 185–86
David, Jacque Louis: *La Mort de Marat,* 147
Davis, Wade, 3, 4, 155
Dawn of the Dead (Romero film), 59, 82–83, 160
Day of the Dead (Romero film), 59, 161
DC Comics, 27–28, 29, 68, 123
Dead City (McKinney), 123
Dead Eyes Open (Shepherd and Boney), 33–37, 35
Deadpool (*Night of the Living Deadpool* character), 29–30
death. *See also* extermination
    attitudes toward, 148
    bioethical issues and definitions of, 175–77
    decay process, 152
    definitions, 152
    geriatric zombies and lack of, ramifications, 19–20, 24, 32, 34
    human body's constant process of, 152–53
    illnesses associated with, 105–6
    inevitability of, 119
    infecting life and cancer's chemicals, 105, 106, 107, 111–14, 115–16, 120
    lack of, as utopian fantasy, 34–35
    life extension as walking, 6
    liminality between life and, 108, 109, 111, 113, 158–59, 163–64, 191, 197
    as normative state, 197
    preference for, 21, 30
death penalty, 63
Death with Interruptions (Saramago), 18
decomposition. *See* body degeneration
Defoe, Daniel, 57
De Humani Corporis Fabrica (Vesalius), 179–80, 182
dehumanization. *See also* medical gaze; nonhumans; Otherness
    of anorexia side effects, 191–92, *192, 193*
    art style techniques representing, 134

bureaucratic social control and herd mentality of, 86–87
human *vs.* nonhuman classifications, 172, 175–76, *176*
of medical school students, 87–91
of patients, 2–3, 21, 33, 36, 76, 126, 137–40
Deleuze, Gilles, 149, 165
dementia, 20, 21–22, 24, 26, 31, 36
demon possession, 27, 201
Dendle, Peter, 86
depression, 2–3, 20
desensitization, 48, 50
desomorphine, 3
detachment. *See* medical gaze
Diagnostic and Statistical Manual of Mental Disorders (DSM), 41, 50, 52
Diane Dillisch (*Revival* character), 33
digital technology, 48, 50, 171, 181, 182–85
disability, 18–19, 23–24, 25–26, 33–36, 205
"(Dis)assembled" (Pfau), 161
dissection
    bioethical definitions of death to justify, 175–76
    corpses as medical school anatomical models for, 146, 151, 153–54, 160
    pathological anatomy experimentation, 171–72, 175–83, *180, 181*
La dissection des parties du corps humain (Estienne and Rivière), 159, *160*
Doctor's Dilemma, The (Shaw), 39, 41
Doctors Without Borders (Médecins Sans Frontières), 68
Donovan, Courtney, 131
Dracula (Stoker), 64
drugs. *See also* chemotherapy
    antibiotics, 41, 61
    cancer, 115
    ethnobiological research on, 3
    for life extension, 6
    with long-term consequences, 62
    with zombie-like side effects, 2–3, 4
DSM (*Diagnostic and Statistical Manual of Mental Disorders*), 41, 50, 52
Dumit, Joseph, 8, 170, 179, 184–85, 186

East End (London), 57, 64
Ebola virus, 63, 68, 124, 137, 140
Eckert, Alissa, 140n2. *See also Preparedness 101: Zombie Pandemic* (Silver, et al.)

Green, Justin, 203
Green, Katie. See *Lighter Than My Shadow* (Green, K.)
"Grey" (Cohen), 151–52
Grey's Anatomy: Raising Hope (television episode), 21
Griffiths, Gareth, 68
Groot, Jerome de, 54, 68
Grosz, Elizabeth, 64–65
Guantanamo, 197
Guattari, Félix, 149, 165

Hagens, Gunther von: *Body Worlds*, 147, 157
Haines, Nikkole: "A Call to Prayer," 96, 96–98, 97, 98, 100
hair loss, 107, 114, 164, 192, 193
Haiti, 4, 7, 79, 133, 165
Halperin, Victor, 59, 79
Halpern, Jody, 93
Hamilton, Sheryl, 139
Happy Zombie Sunrise Home, The (Atwood and Alderman), 26
Haraway, Donna, 109, 179
Harman, Graham, 147–48, 149, 150, 151
hauntic zombies, 106, 108, 109, 119
healthcare
    capitalism and, 196
    class-based access to, 55, 56–57, 64–67, 68–69
    classification based treatment eligibility, 42–47, 44, 45, 46, 50
    geriatric crisis and policy changes in, 20
    health insurance requirements for access to, 68–69, 108
health insurance, 20, 41, 52, 68–69, 108
Heidegger, Martin, 148–49, 150
Helix (television series), 124
Helle, Anita, 204
Hershel (*Walking Dead* character), 24, 46, 47
Herskovits, Elizabeth, 21–22
herstories, 205–7. See also *Lighter Than My Shadow* (Green, K.)
Hirsch (*28 Days Later* comic character), 134, 135, 138
Hirst, Damien, 157
historical narratives. See *New Deadwardians, The*
history, as Otherness, 54
"History of Medical Illustration" (Loechel), 153

hive mentality, 117
Hobbs, Bob, 140n2. See also *Preparedness 101: Zombie Pandemic* (Silver, et al.)
Holmes, Jason: "Being a Patient Made Me a More Empathic (Future) Doctor," 93–94, 94
Holocaust, 35, 192, 194–96, 197, 202
homelikeness, 200
homogenization, 86–87
hordes
    bureaucratic social control descriptions, 86–87
    cancer-causing socialization additions and hive mentality, 117
    of geriatric zombies, 19
    indigenous populations descriptions, 58
    medical student experiences as bureaucratic herd, 86–91
    zombie descriptions, 41, 43, 58, 60, 86
Hottentot Venus, 147
Hughes, Julian C., 21, 36
humanity
    communication skills, 18–19, 24–29, 32–26
    disaster response and loss of, 80
    medical student empathy erosion and loss of, 93–94
    medical student herd and loss of, 86
    neurobiology and brain function for, 177
    vampires and loss of, 62–63
    zombie lack of, 41, 47, 48, 50, 52
humanoids (*Zombie Autopsies* zombie-like characters)
    bioethical issues and ethically dead classifications, 172, 175–78, 176
    brain studies of, 171, 177–83, 180
    descriptions of, 175, 178
humans. See also public response
    brain-dead, and life support debates, 106
    brain-dead, and organ harvesting, 96, 96–99, 97, 98, 176, 177
    injured hands of, 46
    medical interventions and transformations of, 55, 56–57, 60–63
    nonhuman comparisons and desensitization of, 48, 49, 52
    nonhuman comparisons and healthcare eligibility determinations, 42–47, 44, 45, 46
    physiological regeneration of, 152–53

chemical regimes of, 106, 111, 113–14, 116, 119–20
definitions of, 172, 178–79
geriatric zombies and extension of, 6, 19–20, 24, 32, 34
liminality between death and, 108, 109, 111, 113, 158–59, 163–64, 191, 197
Life after Beth (Baena film), 37n5, 55, 191
Lighter Than My Shadow (Green, K.)
    illness and capitalism, 196
    illness and dehumanization effects, 191–94, 192, 193
    illness progression and embodiment descriptions, 198, 199, 200–202
    narrative descriptions, 190, 198
    Obsessive Compulsive Disorder, 199, 203
    self-reflection for rehabilitation and redemption, 202, 205, 210, 212–14, 213
    witnessing process, 195, 196, 203–10, 208, 209, 211
    writing context, 196–97
    zombie narrative comparisons, 191, 210
Lightman, Sarah, 205–6
living dead, the
    brain-dead humans and life support debates, 106
    brain-dead patients and organ harvesting, 96, 96–99, 97, 98
    dementia patients as, 21, 36, 76
    elderly patients as, 36
    global capitalism rethinking, 196
    vampirism as, 55–57, 60–66
Lock, Margaret, 177, 196
Loechel, William, 153
London (Britain), 57, 60, 64–65
loneliness, 80–82
Lord of the Rings, The (Tolkien), 97
love, ethics of, 25–26, 32–36
"Loveliness of Decay, The" (Stommel), 152
Lucy, Saint, 160

mad cow disease. *See* bovine spongiform encephalopathy
magic, as zombie origins theory, 5, 58, 59, 79, 174
Major West (*28 Days Later* character), 133
management models. *See also* containment; extermination
    care and treatment for, 24–26, 28, 46–47

as chronic health condition, 33–36
containment/institutionalization, 32, 33, 35
family/community support, 30–36
medical interventions for human transformation, 55, 56–57, 60–62
Manco, Leonardo, 124
Mann, Sally, 147
mapping, 66
Marchetto, Marisa Acocella: *Cancer Vixen*, 114–16, 120
Marion, Isaac, 123
Marks, J. Ryan, 126–27, 130
martial law, 126, 131, 136
martyrdom, 63, 146, 150, 151, 157, 160
Marvel Zombies (Kirkman and Phillips), 28–29, 123
Matheson, Richard, 156
Mbembe, Achille, 13, 36
McAlister, Elizabeth, 155–56
McCloud, Scott, 170, 200, 204
McGlotten, Shaka, 10n5
McKinney, Joe, 123
Médecins Sans Frontières, 68
medical education. *See also* medical student zombie metaphor comics
    corpses as anatomical models for, 146, 151, 153–54, 160
    supervisors during, 87 91, 88, 89, 90, 91, 92, 94, 101–2
medical gaze
    autopsies and objectivity, 177–78, 182, 183
    body as person *vs.* object, 162, 163–64
    graphic medicine and experience of illness *vs.*, 7, 126–27, 131
    medical student detachment and patient objectification, 95–99, 96, 97, 98
    medical visuality and brain imaging, 178–79
    pathological anatomy and development of, 171–72, 175
medical illustrations
    of anatomy in history, 156, 179, 181, 181–82
    of corpses in history, 153–54, 160, 160–61, 162, 167n10–11
    of fictional zombie autopsies, 179–83, 180
    as Zombie Objects, 153–54
    of zombies, 154, 156–61, 157, 158, 159, 161
"Medical Student: A Tragic Comedy" (Pitzer), 87, 90

medical student zombie metaphor comics
    antisocial behavior themes, 81, 84, 86
    benefits of, 76–77, 99–100, 100–102, 101
    bureaucratic herd associations and dehu-
        manization themes, 87–91, 88, 89, 90,
        91, 92
    consumption themes, 82, 83, 83–86, 84, 85
    empathy erosion themes, 93–94, 94
    environmental context descriptions, 80
    isolation and loneliness themes, 80–82, 81
    medical school comic courses producing,
        77–79
    patient commodification and detachment
        themes, 95–99, 96, 97, 98, 100
    survival themes, 80, 99
medications. See drugs
Merleau-Ponty, Maurice, 149
military culture. See also war
    cancer experience as war metaphor, 110,
        111, 115–16, 120
    color symbolism, 65–66
    disease control and violence legitimization,
        125, 126, 131, 132, 134, 136, 139, 140–
        41n3
    genocidal solutions, 33, 35
    medical interventions as weapons, 61, 67
Miller, Nancy K., 127
Mom's Cancer (Fies), 116–19, 117, 118
Mona and the Little Smile (Burdock), 205
Moore, Lisa Jean, 10n5
Moore, Tony, 44. See also Walking Dead, The
        (Kirkman, Moore, T. and Adlard
        comic)
"Morbific Ensemble" from Soldier's Heart
        (Tyler), 112–13, 113
"Morgue" series (Serrano), 147
Mort de Marat, La (David), 147
Morton, Tim, 147, 148
multiple sclerosis, 18, 20, 22
Mulvihill, Patricia, 65
Murphy, Michelle, 106, 108, 109, 111
Muselmann, 192, 196, 197–98, 210
Mustargen (mustard gas), 106
"My First Big Case" (Lee), 81, 81, 82, 87, 91

Nancy, Jean-Luc, 196
Narcisse, Clairvius, 155
National Geographic (journal), 6–8
national security, 35, 126, 136–37

necrosis, 3
Nekron (Blackest Night character), 27
Nelson, Michael Alan, 124. See also 28 Days
        Later (Nelson, et al. comic)
Neulasta, 115
"Neural Parasitology" (Journal of Experimental
        Biology issue), 4
Neuro (Rose and Abi-Rached), 171, 185
neurobiology
    death definitions and nonhuman classifica-
        tions, 175–77
    drug side effects, 2–3, 4
    humanity distinctions and cognitive func-
        tion, 177
    neurodegeneration, 26, 30, 173–78, 183,
        187n6, 194
    parasitology and, 4–6, 174
New Deadwardians, The (Abnett and Culbard)
    color symbolism, 65–66
    geographic zones and disease associations,
        57, 64–65, 66
    medical intervention and medical misuse
        themes, 55, 56–57, 60–63, 67–68
    series description, overview, 55, 56–57
    social class themes, 55–57, 59, 60–66, 67
    zombiism in, descriptions, 55, 57–59, 60, 67
Newland, Paul, 57, 64, 65
Night of the Living Dead (Romero film), 7, 23,
        52–53n2, 59, 80
Night of the Living Deadpool (Marvel), 29
9/11 attacks, 123, 138
nitrogen mustard (chemical gas), 106
No Longer Human (NLH/Stage IV zombie
        classification), 172, 175, 175–77
nonhumans. See also dehumanization; Other-
        ness
    body degeneration creating, 42
    cognitive function classifications, 28–29,
        41, 47, 48, 50, 52
    healthcare eligibility determinations and
        categorization of, 40–47, 44, 45, 46
    postmodern digital desensitization and
        response to, 48, 50
    sick humans compared to, 139–40
    social class of, 55, 57, 60
    viral infection comparisons, 42
    zombie disease progression and classifica-
        tion as, 134, 172, 175–78, 176
Noomin, Diane, 205–6

Norton, Mike: *Revival,* with Seeley, 30–33, *31*
Notebook, The (Cassavetes book/film), 21

Obamacare, 20, 60, 108
O'Bannon, Dan, 158
objective detachment. *See* medical gaze
object-oriented ontology (OOO), 147–52

obscurity (visual strategy), 26, 30–31, 134
Obsessive Compulsive Disorder (OCD), *199,* 203
Occupy movement, 69
Oleksicki, Marek, 124
Olympic Games, 65
ontic (real) zombies, 106, 108, 119
Ontleding des menschelyken lichaams (Bidloo), 153, *155,* 156
ontologies
    object-oriented (OOO), 147–52
    zombie-oriented (ZOO), 151–52
    zombiism as, 23, 47, 172
"Open Up a Few Brains" from *Neuro* (Rose and Abi-Rached), 171
"Open Up a Few Corpses" from *Birth of the Clinic* (Foucault), 171–72
Ophiocordyceps unilateralis, 4–5
oppression, 32–33, 36, 68, 106, 108, 147, 198, 212
organ harvesting, *96,* 96–99, *97, 98,* 176, 177
Ostherr, Kirsten, 9
Otherness. *See also* dehumanization; non-humans
    anorexia dehumanization as, 194, 212
    cancer and cancer chemicals as, 107–9, *109, 110, 111–12,* 115, 116, 120
    colonialism and perception of, 58–59
    ethnicity as, 132–33
    gender and, 212
    health insurance access limitations as, 108
    history as, 54
    oppression of, 108
    social class of, 56, 57, 59, 60, 64
    terrorists as, 137
    violence legitimization toward, 17
    zombies as, 57
Outbreak (Petersen film), 132
outbreak narratives, 4–8. *See also* viruses and viral epidemics

pandemics. *See* viruses and viral epidemics
"Parasitic Manipulation of Hosts' Phenotype; or, How to Make a Zombie" (*Journal of Integrative and Comparative Biology* issue), 4
parasitology, 4–8, 174
Parkinson's disease, 18, 20, 22
Passage (film), 3
Pasteur, Louis, 57
pathological anatomy, 171–72, 175–83, *180, 181*
pathology research, 57, 58, 59, 173
patients
    cancer, 105, *105,* 116–17, *118*
    civil rights issues and treatment of, 32, 33, 35, 126, 139–40
    dehumanization of, 2–3, 21, 36, 76, 137–40
    extermination of, as murder, 140
    medical gaze and objectification of, 95–99, *96, 97, 98,* 172
    visual imagery assisting, 9
    zombie disease progression and nonhuman classifications, 134, 172, 175–78, *176*
    zombie metaphors for, 127, 128–29, 130
"Penetrated Core (Continued Functioning?)" (Pfau), 160–61, *161*
Peppino, Pablo, 124
personality alterations, 4, 18, 20, 26, 27, 29, 174
"Perspective" (Banbury), 87, *88,* 90–91, *91*
Petersen, Wolfgang, 132
Pfau, George
    art subject and theme descriptions, 161–64, 166–67n9
    "(Dis)assembled," 161
    "Trace" series, 164–65
    "Zombieindex.us," 155–56, 163–64, *163* (detail)
    "Zombie Medical Drawings" series, 154, 156–63, *157, 158, 159, 161,* 165
    "Zombiescapes," 156, 160, 165
pharmaceuticals. *See* drugs
Philippines, 58
Phillips, Sean: *Marvel Zombies,* with Kirkman, 28–29
Pitzer, Michael: "Medical Student: A Tragic Comedy," 87, *90*
Platts, Todd, 190–91
Pokornowski, Steven, 52–53n2
Policing the Crisis (Hall, et al.), 125–26
Polley, Sarah, 21

SARS (severe acute respiratory syndrome), 58, 63, 69n2
Saunders, Lesley, 212
schizophrenia, 4
Schlozman, Steven C., 169. See also *Zombie Autopsies*
science and technology studies (STS), 2, 8–9, 170
Seeley, Tim: *Revival*, with Norton, 30–33, *31*
segregation
    healthcare system based on, 40
    management models based on, 24, 25, 32, 33, 35
    social class, 57, 60, 62, 64
    viral infections and healthcare eligibility determinations, 42–47
Selena (*28 Days Later* character), 133–34, 136, 138, 139
self (I, ego)
    anorexia and perceptions of, 191–92, 194, 200–202, 212, 214
    cancer chemicals and transformation of, 107–9, 110, 114, 115–16, 118
    corpse as absence of, 110
    human matter loss and concept of, 164 65
    life definitions and somatic, 178
    wartime trauma and transformation of, 134, 136, 140–41n3
    zombiism and loss of, 21, 30
Self, Will, 153–54
self-awareness/recognition, 21, 29–30
"Self Replacing Body Trace (Froth)" (Pfau), 164, 165
"Self Replacing Body Trace (Meniscus)" (Pfau), 164
"Self Replacing Body Trace (Pores)" (Pfau), 164
"Self Replacing Body Trace (Slough)" (Pfau), 164
senility (dementia), 20, 21–22, 24, 26, 31, 36
Sensual Object, 147–48
sentience, 18, 25–26, 29–30, 48, 93–94, 194
Serpent and the Rainbow, The (Davis), 3, 155
Serrano, Andres, 147
sexuality, 27, 63, 68, 201–2
Shalvey, Declan, 124
Shaun of the Dead (Wright film), 22–23, 25, 123, 191

Shaw, George Bernard, 39, 41
Shelley, Mary, 54, 59
Shepherd, Matthew: *Dead Eyes Open*, with Boney, 33–37, *35*
shopping malls, 82
Sick Rose, The (Burnett), 153–54
Silver, Maggie, 140n2. See also *Preparedness 101: Zombie Pandemic* (Silver, et al.)
Sims, Bennett: *Questionable Shape, A*, 123
Singer, Merrill, 108–9
slavery
    colonial, 133, 165
    parasitology as, 4–6, 174
    zombie folklore, 5, 79, 174
sleep deprivation, 34, 82
smoking, 116–19, *117*, *118*
Snow, John, 66
social class
    in Edwardian England, 56
    geographical zones and, 57, 64–65, 66
    life worthiness determinations, 137
    lower and working class designations, 56, 57, 64
    medical intervention access based on, 55, 56, 66
    modern healthcare access restrictions due to, 68
    poor/lower working class designations, 55, 57, 59, 60, 67
    and social order reconstruction, 34–36, 55
    as theme, 55–57, 59
    upper/middle aristocracy designations, 55, 56–57, 60, 64, 66
social control, 61, 86–87
sociality, 114–19
Soderbergh, Steven, 131
Soldier's Heart (Tyler), 110–14, *112*, *113*
solitude, 80–82, *81*. See also alienation
somatic self, 178
Sontag, Susan, 194
sound effects, 45–46, *46*, 133–36, *135*
Sparacio, Andrea. See *Zombie Autopsies*
Spinoza, Benedictus de, 121n2
Squier, Susan, 6, 126–27, 130
Squillante, Christian, 83, *83*
"Stage I – Stage II – Stage III – Stage IV" from *Zombie Autopsies*, 175–76, *176*
Stanford School of Medicine, 152–53
Stanley, Wendell M., 140n1

Undead of Alive (film), 123
United States
    aging demographics and birth rate, 19
    colonialism and disease associations, 58
    imperialism and military culture themes, 132
    medical knowledge dissemination criticism, 68
    social class and healthcare access restrictions, 68, 108
universal health care, 40

vaccinations, 50, 61
Valverde de Amusco, Juan, 153, *154*, 156
vampirism
    color symbolism, 65–66
    consequences of, 62–63
    extermination methods, 62
    medical intervention as zombie management model, 55–57, 60–62
    physical descriptions and behaviors, 63
    social class designation, 55, 56–57, 60, 64
    zombie comparisons, 62
Vertigo (DC Comics imprint), 63, 68, 123
Vesalius, Andreas, 156, 179–80, 182
"Victorian Social Body and Urban Cartography, The" (Gilbert), 66
video viruses, 48
violence. *See also* extermination
    cognitive alterity and calculation of, 41, 48, 50, 52
    as geriatric behavior, 20
    physical masking systemic, 43
    public panic and military legitimization of, 125, 131, 132, 136, 139
    as zombie narrative theme, 17, 29–32, 33, 123, 176
Virchow, Rudolph, 57
viruses and viral epidemics
    CDC emergency preparation guidelines for, 3, 76, 124–30, 134
    characteristics of, 39, 124
    geographic zoning and medical mapping practices for, 66
    healthcare economic sustainability issues and treatment eligibility, 40–52, *44*, *45, 46*
    parasitology and, 4–8, 10n6
    public response to, 125–26, 131, 134, 136, 138, 140

technological analogies to, 48
war analogies, 132–34, 135
zombie narrative omissions and assumptions about, 42
zombie narratives with, 139–40
as zombie outbreak narratives, 5, 21, 42, 55, 57, 124, 173–74
vivisections, 175
voodoo, 5, 79, 174

Wald, Priscilla
    disease emergence and racism, 69n2, 132–33
    imperialist attitudes, 134, 137
    outbreak narrative theory, 5
    social order reconstruction, 55, 58
    urban spaces and contagion, 65
    virus characteristics, 140n1
Walking Dead, The (Kirkman, Moore, T. and Adlard comic)
    epidemiological narrative, 23, 40–42, 47, 121n1, 172
    healthcare economic sustainability and exclusion determinations, 42–47, *44*, *45, 46*
    plot descriptions, 43
    television adaptation, 123
    themes, 23, 93
Walking Dead, The (television series)
    geriatric conditions and comparisons, 23–24
    isolation/loneliness imagery, 81
    plot descriptions, 25
    popularity of, 123
    viral epidemic and patient dehumanization, 139–40
Walton, Priscilla, 139
Waples, Emily, 127, 205
war. *See also* military culture
    bioterrorism, 136, 137, 139
    cancer chemicals and metaphors of, 110, 111, 115–16, 120
    on drugs, 3, 35
    media depictions shaping legitimacy of violence, 132–33
    zombie narratives and politics of, 133–34, 136, 139, 140n3
Warm Bodies (Marion novel/Levine film), 25–26, 36, 55, 123, 191

TYPESET BY
Coghill Composition Company

PRINTED AND BOUND BY
Sheridan Books

COMPOSED IN
Minion Pro and Futura

PRINTED ON
50# Natures Natural